Paranasal Sinuses Anatomy and Conditions

Edited by Balwant Singh Gendeh

Published in London, United Kingdom

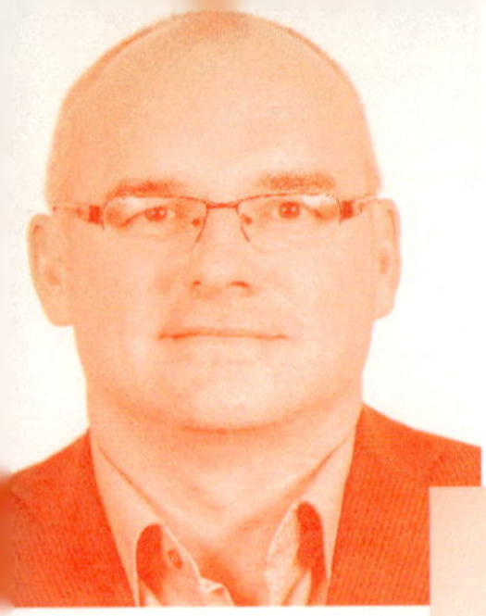
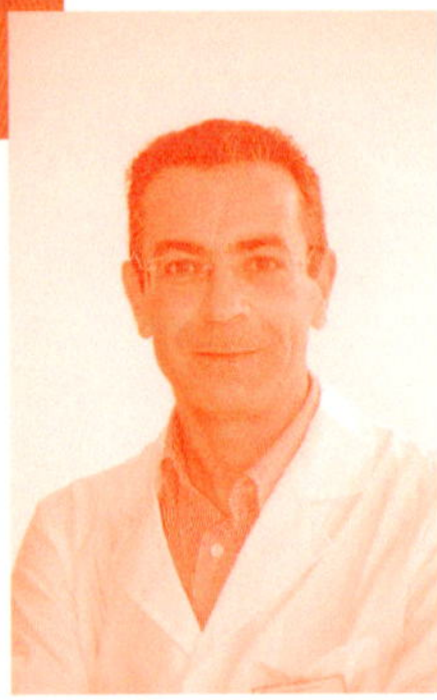
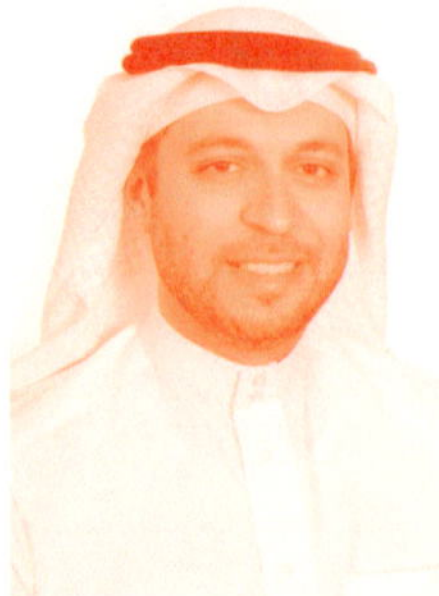
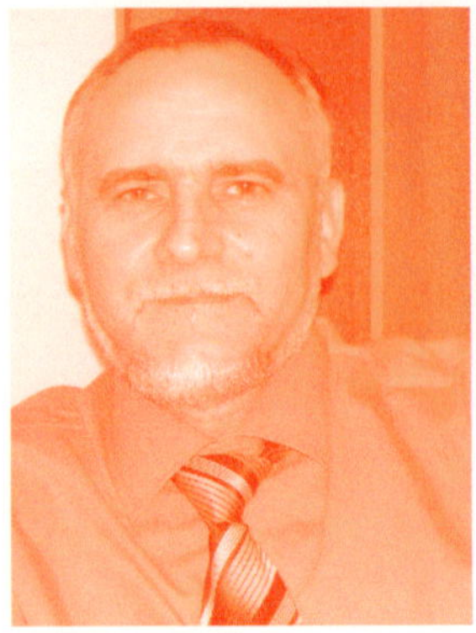
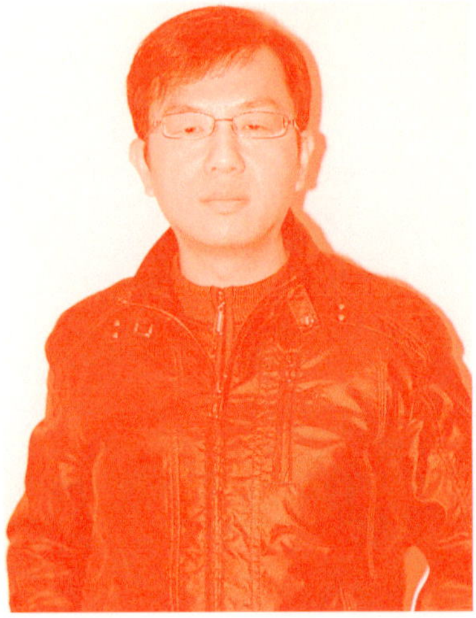
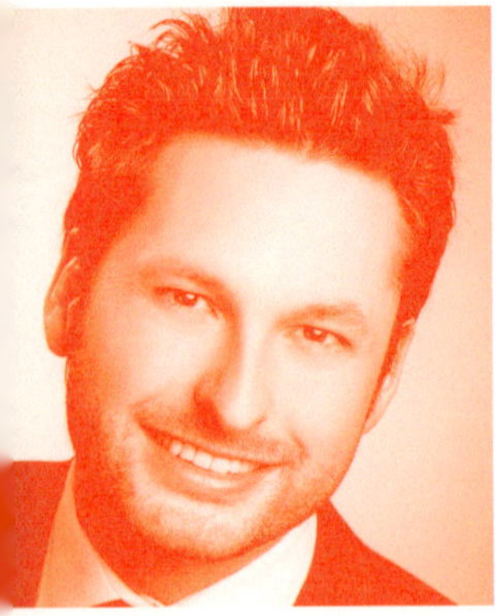
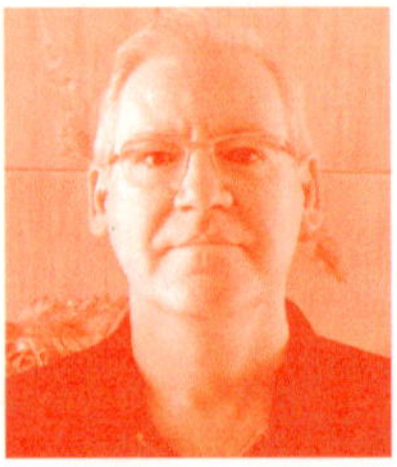

IntechOpen

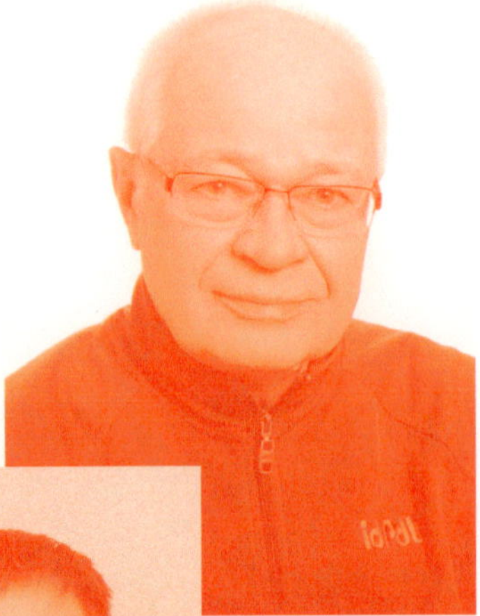
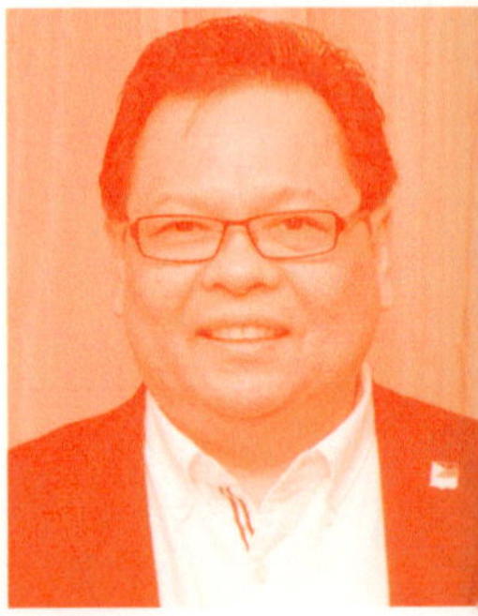
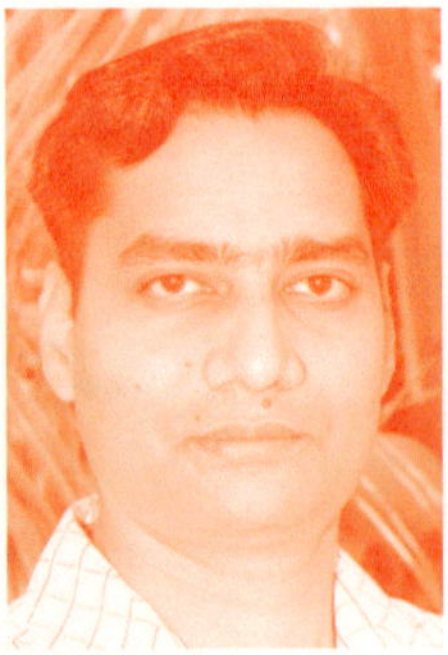
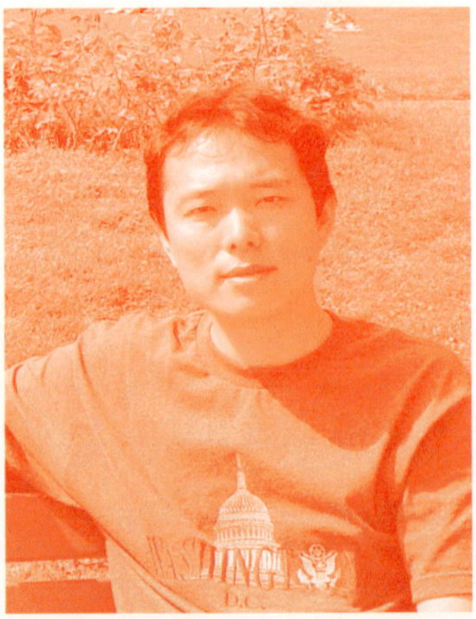
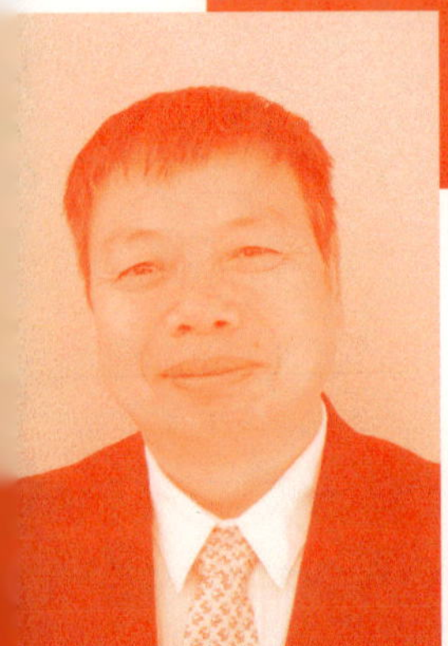
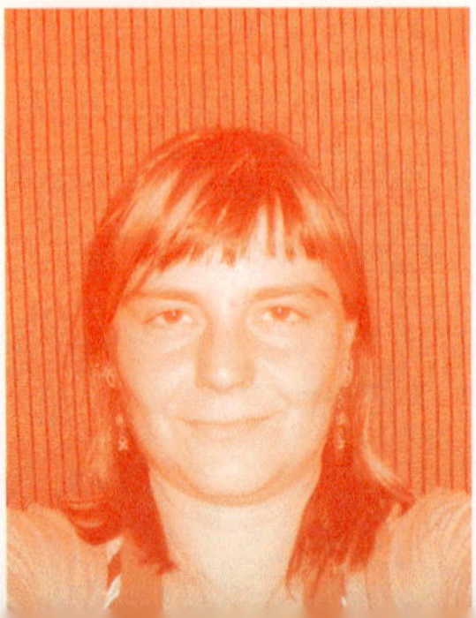

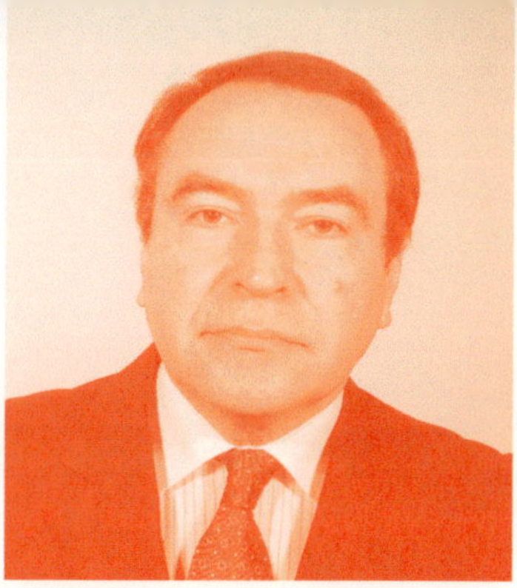
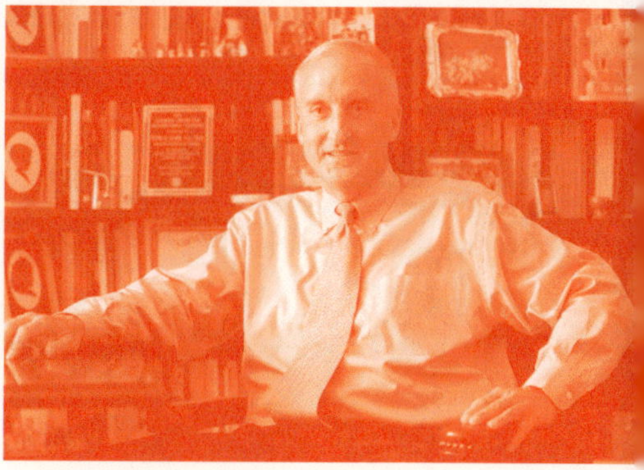
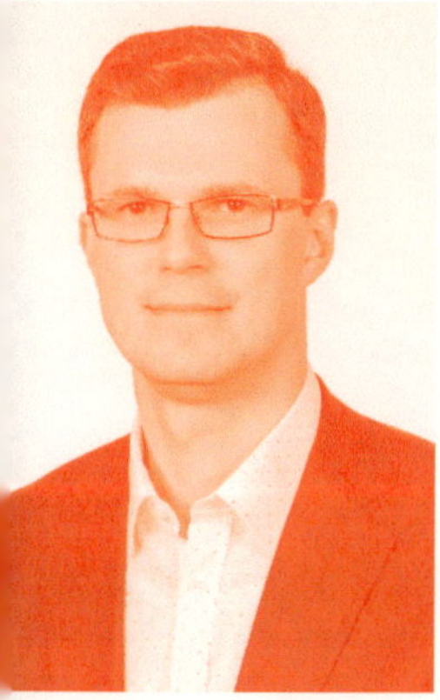
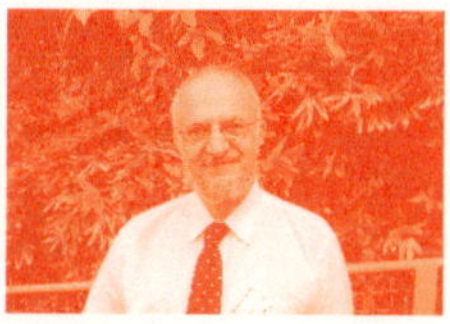
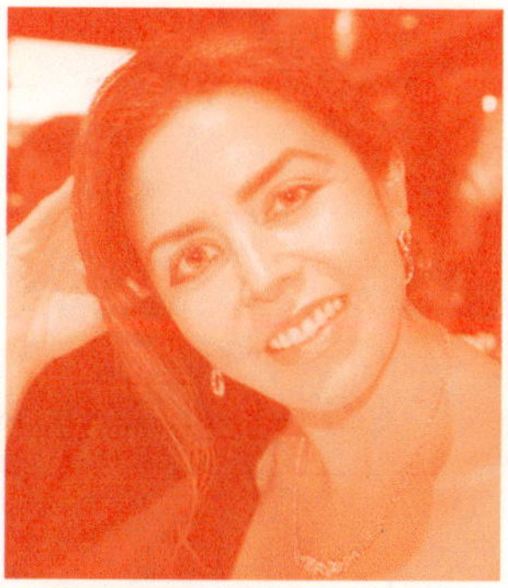

Supporting open minds since 2005

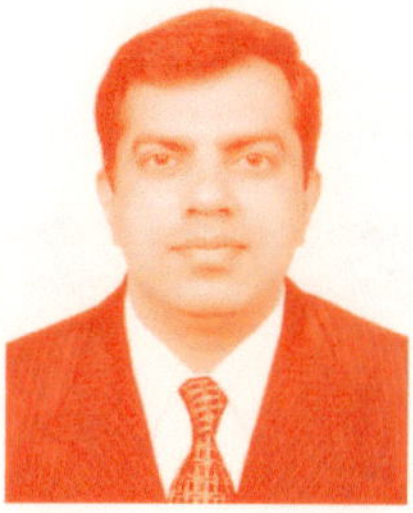
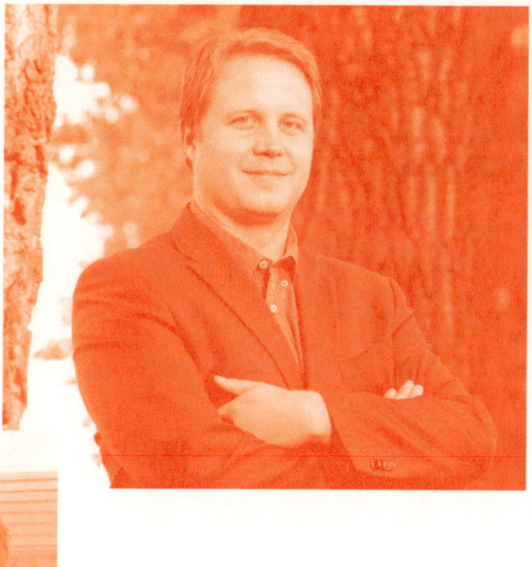
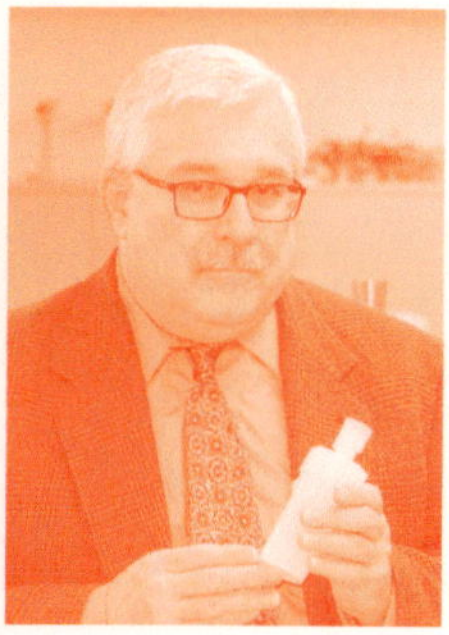
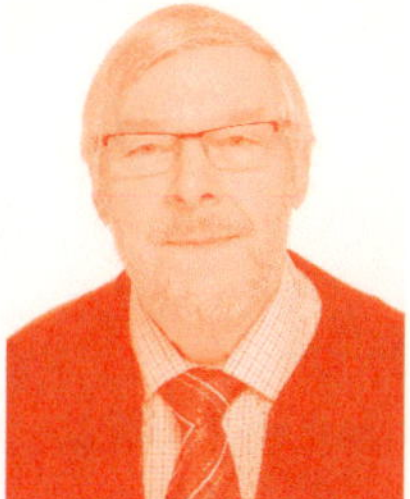
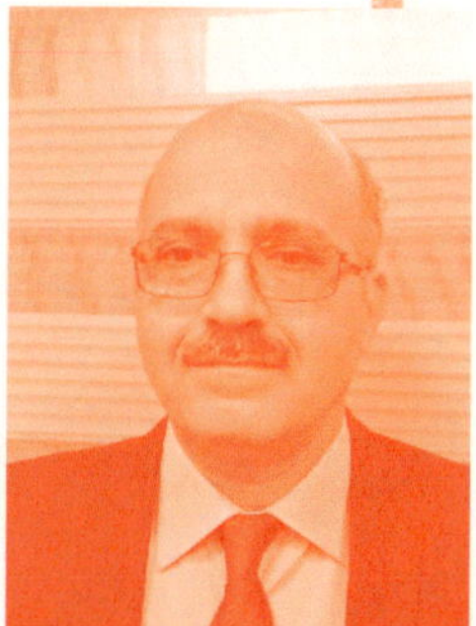
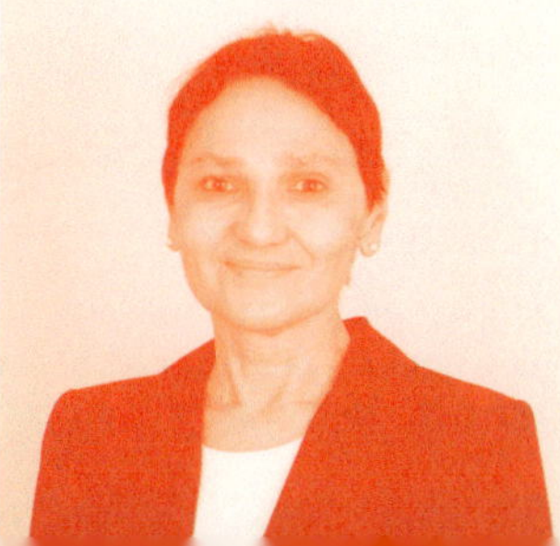
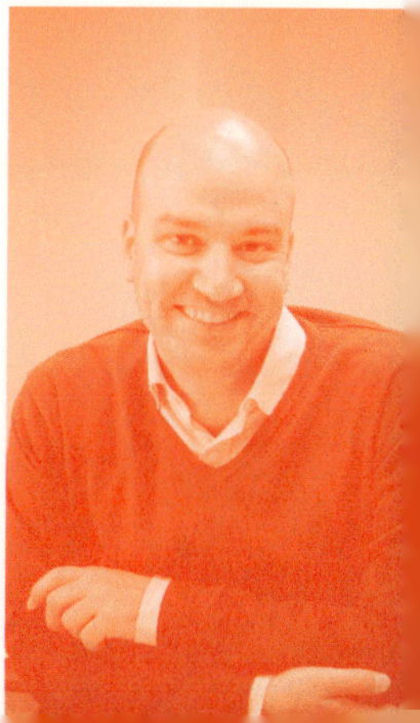

Paranasal Sinuses Anatomy and Conditions
http://dx.doi.org/10.5772/intechopen.94697
Edited by Balwant Singh Gendeh

Contributors
Smail Kharoubi, G. Dave Singh, Elena Bozhikova, Nikolay Uzunov, Jana I. Preis, Anna W. Maro, Sophie Hurez, Sneha Pusapati, Balwant Singh Gendeh, Hardip Singh Gendeh

First published in London, United Kingdom, 2022 by IntechOpen
IntechOpen is the global imprint of INTECHOPEN LIMITED, registered in England and Wales, registration number: 11086078, 5 Princes Gate Court, London, SW7 2QJ, United Kingdom
Printed in Croatia

British Library Cataloguing-in-Publication Data
A catalogue record for this book is available from the British Library

Additional hard and PDF copies can be obtained from orders@intechopen.com

Paranasal Sinuses Anatomy and Conditions
Edited by Balwant Singh Gendeh
p. cm.
Print ISBN 978-1-83969-689-3
Online ISBN 978-1-83969-690-9
eBook (PDF) ISBN 978-1-83969-691-6

For EU product safety concerns:
IN TECH d.o.o., Prolaz Marije Krucifikse Kozulić 3, 51000 Rijeka, Croatia, info@intechopen.com or visit our website at intechopen.com.

Meet the editor

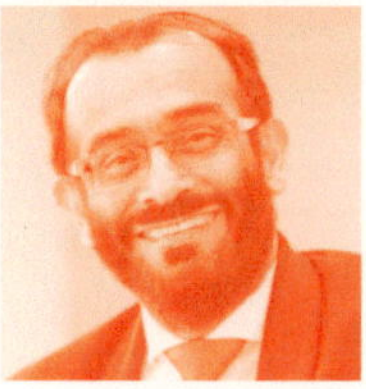

Dr. Balwant Singh Gendeh is a senior consultant ENT surgeon with a sub-specialty interest in rhinology (allergy, sino-nasal diseases, endoscopic sinus, anterior and ventral skull base surgery, and functional and cosmetic nasal surgery). He was an ENT registrar at the Royal Infirmary, Middlesbrough, UK, in 1993, and a JW Fulbright scholar, University of Pittsburgh, USA, in 1997. During his Fulbright experience, he also worked at the Hospital of the University of Pennsylvania (HUP), Philadelphia, USA, and St. Joseph's Hospital, Chicago, USA, with a sub-specialty interest in rhinology and aesthetic nasal surgery. Dr. Gendeh retired after thirty-eight years of government service as a consultant ENT surgeon at the National University of Malaysia Medical Centre (UKMMC) in 2014. Currently, he is a visiting professor at the Department of Otorhinolaryngology-Head and Neck Surgery, UKMMC, and a resident ENT consultant at Pantai Hospital Kuala Lumpur. He is an executive member of numerous national and international bodies including board chairman of the Malaysian American Commission on Educational Exchange (MACEE). He was elected as a diploma of the Fellowship Academy of Medicine Malaysia (FAMM) in 2000, an international fellow of the Academy of Otolaryngology Head and Neck Surgery in 2004, a fellow of the Academy of Sciences Malaysia (FASc) in 2016, and a fellow of Malaysian Scientific Association (FMSA) in 2017. He has written ninety-three scientific papers and edited/co-edited eight books and seven book chapters.

Contents

Preface

This book discusses selected topics on the anatomy of paranasal sinuses and related conditions, providing insight into advancements in the field.

It is divided into two sections: "Rhinology" and "Maxillofacial." The first section covers morphological aspects of the maxillary sinus, infectious causes of acute and chronic sinusitis, posterior ethmoidal artery, and paranasal sinuses anatomy and anatomical variations. The second section covers sinonasal-associated midfacial expansion and maxillary sinus in dental implantology. Chapters present new clinical and research developments as well as future perspectives on ever-expanding upper airway and jaw problems. The book is intended for ENT surgeons, rhinologists, maxillofacial surgeons, postgraduates, researchers, trainees, and general practitioners with a special interest in upper airway diseases.

I would like to thank and congratulate the chapter authors for their excellent contributions.

I would also like to thank the valuable teachers from whom I have gained knowledge throughout the years. I am grateful to IntechOpen for conceiving this book project and for asking me to serve as editor. Thanks also go to Author Service Manager Marica Novakovic at IntechOpen for guiding me through the publication process and moving the book ahead in a timely fashion. My kind gratitude goes to the technical editors for arranging the book in a uniform format. I hope this publication contributes to the global distribution of knowledge of the anatomy of the nose, sinuses, and maxillofacial conditions.

I would like to dedicate this book to my spouse, children, and loved ones for all their patience and understanding.

Balwant Singh Gendeh, MBBS(Kashmir), MS(ORL-HNS), UKM, AM(Mal), FAMM, FASc (M'sia), FMSA
Retired Professor,
Department of ORL-HNS,
UKM Medical Center,
Cheras, Kuala Lumpur

Senior Consultant ENT Resident Surgeon,
(Rhinology -Allergy, Endoscopic Sinus & Skull Base Surgery,
Functional & Cosmetic Nasal Surgery),
Pantai Hospital,
Kuala Lumpur, Malaysia

Section 1

Rhinology

Chapter 1

Morphological Aspects of the Maxillary Sinus

Elena Bozhikova and Nikolay Uzunov

Abstract

The development of modern surgical methods and techniques for treatment of the diseases of the paranasal sinuses and the edentulous ridge of the maxilla requires detailed knowledge of the anatomy, physiology and pathology of the maxillary sinus. The sinus dimensions and volume, thickness of the mucosa, height of the inferior wall and presence of septa and root prominence are important indicators for the pneumatization of the maxillary sinus and have essential role by performing sino-nasal and dental implant surgery. The preliminary assessment of some morphological aspects of the maxillary sinus is essential for the proper diagnosis and treatment of a number of diseases in maxillofacial region, including treatment of the chronic rhinosinusitis and the edentulous ridges of the distal maxilla.

Keywords: anatomy, maxillary sinus, sinus development, sinus walls, sinus septa, sinus mucosa

1. Introduction

A considerable portion of the pathology of the maxillofacial region affects the maxillary sinus (MS). These include various inflammatory processes (rhinogenic, allergic, odontogenic), systemic, endocrinological (Grave's disease) and oncological disease, traumas, congenital anomalies and acquired defects (traumatic, post-resection, etc.), as well as diseases with unclear etiology (silent sinus syndrome).

The close relations of the MS with the nasal and oral cavities, orbit, pterygopalatine and infratemporal fossae are precondition for spreading of pathological processes from the sinus to neighboring areas and vise versa. The ophthalmic symptoms by the silent sinus syndrome are due to proximity between the orbit and the sinus, and the proximity between the floor of the MS and the roots of the upper molars and premolars allows odontogenic infections to induce changes in the sinus mucosa, also acute and chronic sinusitis. The thin or missing bone plate between the dental apex and the floor of the sinus is a factor that can lead to post-extraction hemorrhages, oro-antral communications, luxation of tooth roots and foreign bodies, compression of canal fillers, penetrations of cysts and invasion of tumors in the sinus, etc.

As an important anatomical structure, the maxillary sinus is a subject of various surgical interventions in rhinological, endoscopic, ophthalmic and maxillofacial surgery, and neurosurgery. The main aim of maxillary sinus operations is to preserve its anatomical and functional integrity. This is possible after preoperative assessment of the morphological characteristics of the sinus, such as its volume, linear dimensions, wall thickness, septa, position and permeability of its drainage ostium.

Regeneration of orofacial functions often requires reconstruction of the damaged alveolar process. The reduction of the dento-alveolar segment occurs under the influence of various etiological factors (dental extractions, inflammatory and systemic diseases, traumas, tumors, congenital anomalies). The resulting bone defects disrupt the anatomy, biomechanics and the relations between the two jaws. The quantity of bone loss determines the severity of morphological and functional lesions in the orofacial system – nutrition, speech, breathing, facial expressions, common and specific senses, social contacts. According to this the reconstruction of bone defects and deficits of both jaws has psych-social significance.

Detailed research and modern clinical interpretation of the anatomy, physiology and pathology of the maxillary sinus are an important condition for the development and improvement of modern operative and reconstructive techniques and for the prevention of postoperative complications. This contributes both to regeneration and maintenance of the health and self-esteem of the individual, as well as to his social realization.

2. Development of the maxillary sinus

MS begins its development in the tenth gestation week (GW) by primary pneumatization. It arises from the middle nasal meatus and spreads into the ethmoid cartilage. Initially, a small ridge is formed above the inferior nasal concha, from which *processus uncinatus* develops. The already formed uncinate process of the ethmoid bone grows in medial direction and forms the ethmoid infundibulum. It presents as a groove between the nasal infundibulum and the lateral wall. The mucosa of the anterior wall of the ethmoid infundibulum, lateral to the uncinate process, forms several invaginations in the surrounding mesenchyme. These invaginations form a furrow, named uncibullous groove. During the 11th week a cavity is formed from this furrow, which represents the primary MS [1].

In the 20th gestation week the secondary pneumatization of the sinus begins and spreads within the maxilla. The dimensions of MS increase at different rates during the different periods of the fetal development. The antero-posterior (AP) dimension increases most significantly, being larger in male fetuses [2].

During its development, variations in the shape of the MS are observed due to its growth in different directions, but at the end of the embryonic period it is oval-shaped. In the cavity of the sinus, septa and recesses can be observed, but after the 29th week they disappear. From 10 to 16 GW the floor of the sinus is located above the attachment of the inferior nasal concha, in 17-20th weeks it is at the level of the attachment, and after 21st week - below its level. Ossification is observed for the first time in the lateral wall of the MS in the 16th GW. Subsequently, in the 20th gestation week, it spreads into the anterior wall, and in the 21st week it comprises its posterior wall. Up to 37 GW, the medial wall does not ossify. The drainage ostium of MS is located in the anterior one-third of the ethmoid infundibulum, between processus uncinatus and lamina papiracea. No additional openings are observed during embryonic development. Asymmetry between the sinuses was found in 30% of the cases, but maxillary hypoplasia was absent [3].

The secondary pneumatization of the maxilla begins in the 5th month after birth, and at this stage the MS is presented as a triangular space located medially to the infraorbital foramen. The growth of the sinus slightly precedes the development of the maxilla and is accomplished by resorption of its walls, except the medial one, which plays a role of a depot. The lateral wall of the nasal cavity (NC) is also resorbed, and this leads to its expansion. The lack of resorption in the medial wall of MS prevents the development of an extensive communication between the sinus and the nasal cavity [4].

At birth, the MS presents as a longitudinal furrow filled with fluid. It is found on the medial surface of the maxilla above the germs of the upper first molars. The dimensions of the MS at birth are: length (antero-posterior direction) - 7,3 ± 2,7 mm; height - 4,0 ± 0,9 mm; width - 2,7 ± 0,8 mm. At the age of 16 the dimensions are respectively: length 38,8 ± 3,5 mm; height 36,3 ± 6,2 mm; width 27,5 ± 4,2 mm [4]. It is considered that the growth of the sinus is 2 mm per a year in vertical direction and 3 mm in the antero-posterior direction [5].

At the end of the 1st year the lateral border of the MS is located below the medial part of the orbit, in the 2nd year - it reaches the level of the infraorbital canal, and in the 3rd and 4th years it is located inferolateral to the infraorbital canal [6].

The increase of the MS in height of up to 3 years of age is directly related to the maxilla and depends on several factors such as: the pressure of the eye bulb on the orbital floor; the traction of the maxilla as a result of the action of the facial muscles, the muscles of the soft palate and the muscles attached to the mandible; teeth eruption. After the age of 3, the influence of the eyeball decreases, but the pulling action of the muscles continues, which leads to a growth of the frontal process of the maxilla. The growth of the MS is directly related to the eruption of the upper teeth. At the age of 9 years, the lateral border of the sinus reaches the floor of the nasal cavity [6].

In the 15th year after birth, the lateral growth of the MS stops. In early childhood, its floor is located at the level of the middle nasal meatus; in the 8-9th year - close to the floor of the NC, and in the 12th year it reaches the level of the hard palate. The sinus reaches its final dimensions after the eruption of the third molar [6].

As a result of the rapid development of the MS, its floor after birth is located lower than its drainage opening to the nasal cavity. As the sinus grows, close relationships arise with the roots of the upper molar and premolar teeth. During the eruption of each tooth, its bone bed is occupied by the pneumatic sinus, as a result of which the sinus floor is located initially at the level of the floor of the NC, and subsequently below it. The MS can grow not only between the roots of neighboring teeth, but also between the roots of the same tooth, resulting in their protrusion into the cavity of the sinus. As the MS grows within the maxilla and at its expense, recessions are gradually formed, which are designated as zygomatic, alveolar, infraorbital and palatine.

3. Anatomy of maxillary sinus

The MS is located entirely inside the maxilla and is the largest of the paranasal sinuses. It usually represents a single-chamber cavity, but in some cases two sinuses separated by bone septa can be found. It has a shape of four-walled pyramid with a base located medially to the NC (the lateral wall of the nose) and an apex directed towards the zygomatic arch.

3.1 Dimensions and volume of the maxillary sinus

The size of the sinus varies, and according to literature data, its average dimensions are depth - 34 to 45 mm, width - 25 to 35 mm, height - 33 to 44 mm and volume - 3 to 30 cm^3 (**Figures 1** and **2**).

The highest value of the cranio-caudal dimension in 93% of cases was measured around the second molar, and for the medio-lateral and antero-posterior in 90% of cases - at the level of the root of the zygomatic complex. In females, the size of the MS is smaller. A cadaveric study of 31 semi-heads shows that the height (cranio-caudal dimension) of the MS ranges between 10,98 mm and 39,14 mm (mean - 24,05 ± 6,3 mm); the antero-posterior dimension - between 14,27 mm and 42,09 mm (mean - 28,65 ± 7,2 mm), and the medio-lateral dimension - between

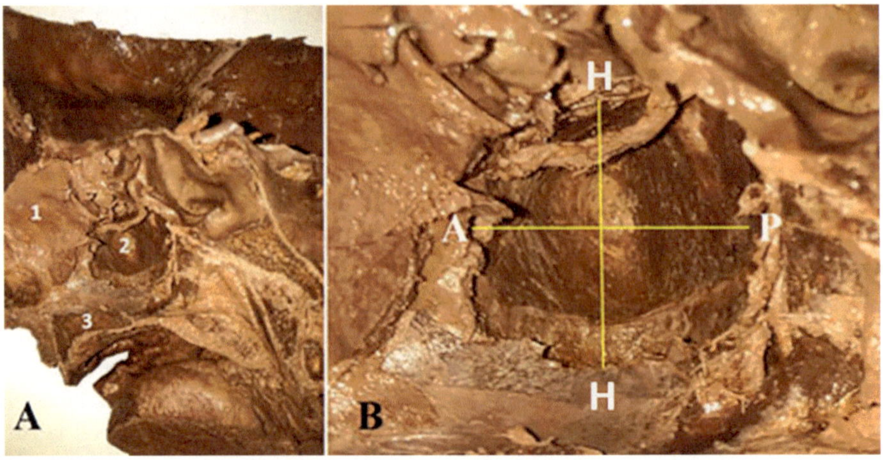

Figure 1.
Schematic representation of the antero-posterior (A–P) dimension and the height (H) of the MS on cadaveric head with medial access: A. sagittal section of cadaveric head (1 – Nasal septum; 2 – мaxillary sinus; 3 – Hard palate); B. maxillary sinus on the same cadaveric head (A-P – Antero-posterior dimension; H – Height).

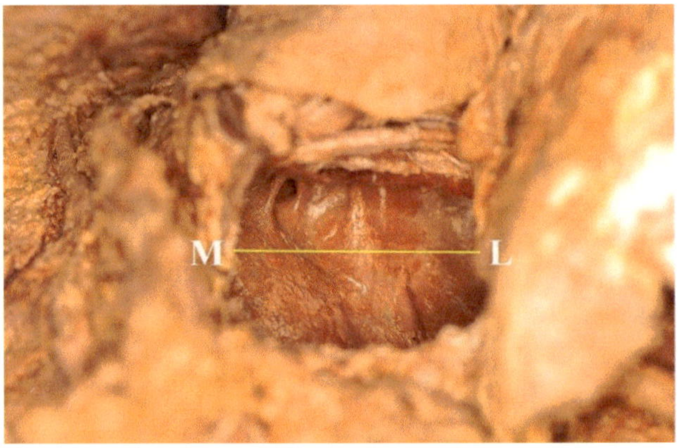

Figure 2.
Schematic representation of the medio-lateral dimension (M-L) of the MS on cadaveric head with anterior access.

11,38 mm and 36,19 mm (mean - 20,08 ± 5,04 mm). This study reveals that the medio-lateral dimension is the smallest. The volume of the MS ranges between 4,00 and 19 cm^3. The average volume of the sinus is 11,7 ± 3,98 cm^3 [7].

3.2 Walls of the maxillary sinus

3.2.1 Medial wall

From a surgical point of view, the medial wall can be divided in two parts: a lower one, called a "surgical" wall, which corresponds to the inferior nasal meatus and is bounded superiorly by the tuberosity of the inferior nasal concha, and inferiorly - by the floor of the nasal cavity; and upper, called "physiological", located in the middle nasal meatus, and enclosed between the inferior and middle nasal concha. In the surgical part the sinus hiatus is found, which is extremely easily fractured and is bounded by the frontal and palatine processes of the maxilla. Here is also located the crest of the inferior nasal concha [8].

The medial wall of the MS has a quadrangular shape and corresponds to the inner (nasal) surface of the maxilla, on which there is a large opening - hiatus maxillaris. It represents the base of the pyramid and is at the same time a lateral wall of the NC. This wall descends below the level of the nasal floor and is attached directly to the palatine process of the maxilla. Its thickness varies in different areas – it is thinnest in the middle of its lower end, and thickest – in its antero-inferior angle. The medial wall has a complex structure, with the nasal conchas lying on the outside. It is formed mostly by the mucosa of the middle nasal meatus, the lining of the MS, and a layer of connective tissue between them. On the side of the NC, the medial wall also includes the inferior nasal meatus and the floor of the nasal fossa.

After removal of the middle nasal concha, the medial wall is composed of bulla ethmoidalis, processus uncinatus and hiatus maxillaris, which has a semi-lunar shape and represents a gap between processus uncinatus (below) and bulla ethmoidalis (above). Hiatus maxillaris is narrowed by several bones. The lacrimal bone is located anteriorly, the labyrinth of the ethmoid bone with the superior and middle nasal concha – superiorly, the perpendicular plate of the palatine bone and the medial plate of the pterygoid process of the sphenoid bone – posteriorly, and below – the ethmoid and lacrimal processes of the inferior nasal concha. Processus uncinatus is a sickle-shaped bone plate that divides the hiatus maxillaris into anterior, posterior, and superior orifices. The upper opening is called hiatus semilunaris. In 1870, Zuckerkandal [9] introduced the term fontanelle. The fontanelle is an area in the middle nasal meatus, located below the uncinate process and above the inferior nasal concha, and covered medially by the nasal mucosa, and laterally - by the mucous membrane of the MS, with connective tissue between them. In this area there is no bone, therefore it is prone to perforation. Depending on their location relative to processus uncinatus, the anterior and posterior fontanelles differ. The anterior fontanelle is located between the lower edge of the uncinate process and the attached edge of the inferior nasal concha, while the posterior one is in postero-superior direction relative to the anterior one. The drainage opening of the MS opens in hiatus semilunaris. The mucosa of processus uncinatus along its upper border is attached loosely to the underlying bone, forming laterally a depression in a shape of a shallow pocket. At the antero-superior end of hiatus semilunaris a funnel-shaped fossa is located called infundibulum ethmoidalis, which extends to the recessus frontalis. The frontal sinus is drained in it.

Ostium maxillare (**Figure 3**) is located in the upper third of the medial sinus wall and drains into the posterior part of the semilunar hiatus in about 52–78% of cases [10]. It has an oval shape and is located in a transverse direction. Its

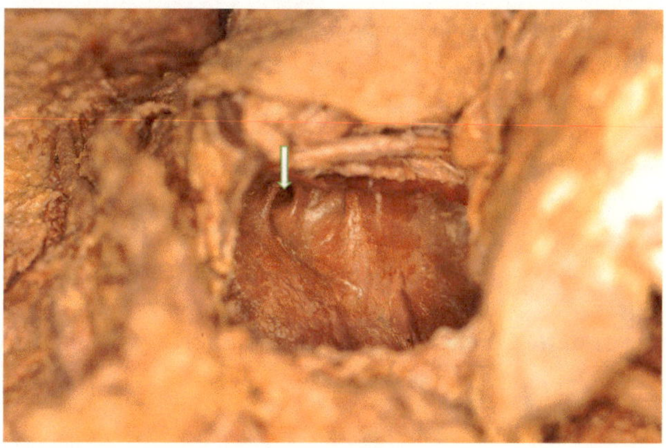

Figure 3.
Medial wall of maxillary sinus with ostium maxillare (arrow).

dimensions range from 1 to 17 mm, on average about 2–4 mm in diameter [11]. The opening is found 18–35 mm superiorly to the floor of the nasal cavity and about 28 mm superiorly to the sinus floor. In women, the distance between the floor of the nasal cavity and the opening is less [12].

Due to the high position of ostium maxillare, the drainage of the MS is difficult and is accomplished due to the active oscillations of the cilia of the epithelium. As a result, infections in the middle nasal meatus can compromise the sinus drainage.

Sometimes additional drainage openings are also found. Their frequency ranges from 0–43% [13]. The size of the openings is from 1 to 10 mm, and their number is variable. They are located in the area of the anterior fontanelle or distal to the natural opening, in the area of the posterior fontanelle [13]. Additional drainage openings can also occur as a result of pathological processes. They are detected in 30% of patients with chronic rhinosinusitis and in 10–20% of healthy individuals [14]. In some cases, ostium maxillare merges with the additional openings and a large drainage opening is formed.

The drainage of the MS occurs only through ostium maxillare, therefore the presence of additional openings can lead to reabsorption of mucus through them [15]. They do not participate in the physiological drainage of the sinus, even if its natural opening is blocked [9].

3.2.2 Superior wall

The superior wall of the MS usually has a triangular shape and represents the orbital surface of the maxilla, which participates in the formation of most of the orbital floor. Its width is greater than that of the inferior wall and is inclined downwards and forwards and laterally. It is extremely thin and fragile, further weakened by the passing sulcus et canalis infraorbitalis, which are located in its middle third and 5–7 mm to 10 mm from the lower orbital border. The canal causes a well-defined bone ridge along the upper wall. It opens on the anterior surface of the maxilla through foramen infraorbitale. The infraorbital nerve-vascular bundle is located in it. Often on some places in the infraorbital canal there is no bone plate and in these cases the nerve-vascular bundle is covered only by the mucous membrane of the sinus. The highest part of the roof of the MS is located below the orbital apex.

3.2.3 Anterior wall

The anterior wall of the MS represents the anterior surface of the maxilla, extending from the inferior orbital margin to the alveolar process, and posteriorly - to zygomaticoalveolar crest. The external surface is covered with soft tissues. On the anterior surface of the maxilla lie the facial artery and vein, lymphatic vessels, motor branches of the facial nerve and sensory branches of the infraorbital nerve. On this wall there is a well-defined depression, called fossa canina, which is located above the root of the upper canine. This is the place with the thinnest cortical plate. The suborbital sulcus is also located on this surface. The cortical plate of the anterior wall thickens at its periphery. On the internal surface of the anterior wall, under the mucosa, the nerve-vascular bundles for the frontal teeth and premolars descend – middle and anterior superior alveolar nerves (branches of the infraorbital nerve), which participate in the formation of superior dental plexus, and anterior superior alveolar arteries and veins.

3.2.4 Posterior (infraorbital) wall

The posterior wall of the MS lies behind the zygomaticoalveolar ridge. It is divided into two sections: medial or pterygomaxillary and lateral or zygomatico-tuberal.

The medial part of the wall is thin, corresponds to the maxillary tuber and behind it are located the infratemporal and pterygopalatine fossae.

The lateral part of the wall is formed by the zygomatic process of the upper jaw with zygomaticoalveolar crest and the surface anterior to the tuber. On this place is also located the intraosseous anastomosis between the infraorbital and posterior superior alveolar artery, which is of great clinical importance in surgical interventions. Some anatomical structures such as the zygomatic wall and maxillary tuberosity can affect the thickness of the lateral wall.

The lateral wall of the sinus increases in thickness from the second premolar to the second molar from 5 to 15 mm. The average thickness of the lateral wall in partially edentulous jaws is 1,71 ± 0,12 mm, while in totally edentulous it was 1,57 ± 0,07 mm [16]. The lateral wall thickness is 1,69 ± 0,71 mm in the area of the first premolar; 1,50 ± 0,72 mm in the area of the second premolar; 1,77 ± 0,78 in the area of the first molar; and 1,89 ± 0,85 mm in the area of the second molar [17].

The height of the residual alveolar ridge, the type of edentulousness (partial or total) and age affect the thickness of the lateral wall. The smaller the residual height of the alveolar ridge is, the lateral wall is thinner [16]. The smaller thickness of the lateral wall also implies lower bone density [18].

3.2.5 Inferior wall (floor)

The inferior wall of the MS is formed by the lateral region of the alveolar process of the maxilla, in which the premolars and molars are located. Its boundaries are usually the first premolar anteriorly and a small recess behind the third molar. The floor of MS in about 63% is located lower than that of the NC, in about 33% it is at the level of the floor of the NC, and in 5–10% - higher [19]. Most often it is located 1.5 cm below the floor of the NC along the horizontal line connecting the lower edges of ala nasi. According to other authors, the sinus floor is located 7–8 mm below the floor of the NC [10].

The shape of the sinus floor is concave (rounded), most often mono- or biconcave. In other cases, the floor of the MS has an irregular or flat shape [20].

The inferior wall is composed of basal and alveolar bone. The alveolar bone consists of cortical plate, which is in contact with the teeth, and spongiosis is located inside.

The floor of the MS is located downwards and laterally to the alveolar ridge of the maxilla, as a result of which recesses may form between the roots of the posterior teeth. An alveolar recess is found in approximately 50% of the maxillary sinuses, which can lead to perforations of the floor during endodontic and surgical treatment.

The roots of the upper lateral teeth are located in close proximity to the floor of the MS. The relationship between the roots of the teeth and the floor of the sinus can be divided into three main groups: distant - there is a thick bone wall between the apices of the dental roots and the sinus floor; tangential - there is a very thin bone plate between the roots and the floor of the MS; and penetrating - the roots of the teeth are covered only by the sinus mucosa. The bony lamella separating the floor of the sinus and the roots of the teeth decreases in thickness from 6,9 mm in canines to 1,7 mm at the second molar, and in the area of the third molar it increases to 2,8 mm [20].

Approximately 78% of the posterior maxillary teeth are located in dangerous proximity to the floor of the MS or protrude into it, which is a prerequisite for the occurrence of various complications during their endodontic treatment or extraction. The protruding roots are usually separated from the sinus with a thin bone plate of varying thickness, and sometimes covered only by a mucous membrane. They form conical elevations on the floor of the sinus. The roots of the first and second molars most often protrude into the cavity of the MS (**Figure 4**).

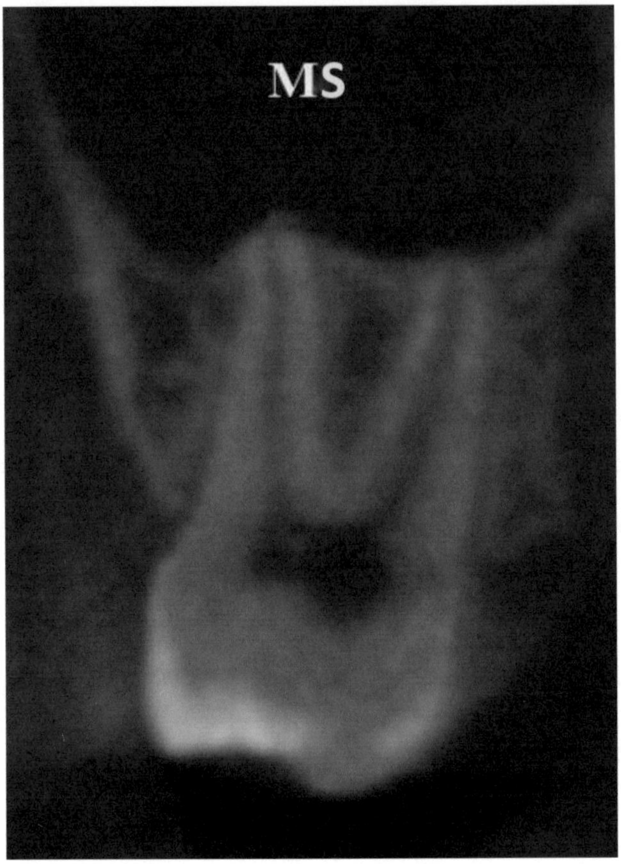

Figure 4.
Protrusion of the mesio-buccal root of upper left second molar in the cavity of the maxillary sinus (MS).

Most of the roots of the first and second premolars (77–98%) are not in close relations with the floor of the MS. In contrast, the roots of molars are in close proximity to the sinus floor: 37% of the first molars, 55% of the second and 31% of the third molars are in close contact with the floor of the MS [21]. The roots of the second molars are located in close proximity to the sinus floor, and most often tangential or penetrating relations are found. In this area is also the lowest point on the floor of the MS [20, 21]. The buccal roots of the second molar protrude most often in the cavity of the MS [22]. Regarding the first molar, the buccal roots most often protrude in the MS, while their palatine roots most often protrude laterally.

There are no statistically significant differences between genders, and the right and left sinus [22–24].

Different classifications of the relationships between the roots of the upper lateral teeth and the floor of the MS have been created in order to predict and avoid possible complications during endodontic, orthodontic and surgical treatment. All modern classifications are based on those created by Freisfeld et al. [25] and Kwak et al. [26].

Freisfeld et al. [25] offer three types of vertical relationships: class 0 - the dental roots of the upper lateral teeth are not in contact with the floor of MS; class 1 - the roots are in contact with the sinus floor, but do not protrude into the sinus cavity; class 2 - the roots of the teeth protrude into the sinus.

In 2004, Kwak et al. [26] classify the relationships between the floor of the MS and the roots of the upper teeth into five classes: class 1 - the floor of MS is located above the line connecting the buccal and palatine root apices; class 2 – the sinus floor is located below the line connecting the buccal and palatine root apices, without the presence of apical protrusion; class 3 - apical protrusion of the buccal root tip above the sinus floor; class 4 - apical protrusion of the palatine root tip above the sinus floor; class 5 - apical protrusion of the buccal and palatine root tips above the sinus floor. The authors also create a classification for the horizontal relationships between the MS floor and the upper lateral teeth. These relations are divided into three classes: class 1 - the alveolar recess of the floor is located to a greater extend in the direction of the buccal wall compared to the buccal root; class 2 - the alveolar recess is located between the buccal and palatine roots; class 3 - the alveolar recess is located to a greater extend in the direction of the palatine wall than the palatine root.

Didilescu et al. [27] offer a classification based on the measured distance between the root apex and the floor of the MS (thickness of the bone plate between the root tip and the sinus floor). The topographic relations between the floor of the sinus and the root apices of the first upper molars are divided into five classes: class 0 – the distance between the root apex and the sinus floor is 0 mm; class 1 - the distance between the root apex and the floor of the MS is between 0 and 2 mm; class 2 - the distance between the root apex and the sinus floor is between 2 and 4 mm; class 3 - the distance between the root apex and the sinus floor is between 4 and 6 mm; class 4 - the distance between the root apex and the sinus floor is greater than 6 mm.

This classification also allows an assessment of the topography of the root furcation relative to the floor of the sinus. In the relationships of the roots of the upper first molar with the floor of MS of class 2, 3 or 4, the lowest mean value of the bone plate between the floor of the sinus and the furcation is 7,64 mm respectively; 9,69 mm; and 12,41 mm These cases favor direct implant placement after tooth extraction without lifting the MS floor. In class 0 and 1, the implementation of endodontic treatment, tooth extraction and immediate placement of dental implants requires special attention.

The close relationships between the apices of the dental roots and the floor of the MS determine the possibility of spreading dental infections to MS and influence endodontic, orthodontic and surgical treatment, as well as the planning and implementation of dental implant treatment.

The tangential and penetrating relations between the roots of the teeth and the floor of the MS are a predisposing factor for the occurrence of various complications during the extraction of upper molars such as oro-antral fistulas or root penetration into the sinus cavity. They are also the cause of various complications during surgical interventions in oral implantology, resulting in development of chronic maxillary sinusitis [20].

3.3 Septa

The septa (**Figure 5**) were first described by Underwood [28, 29] and are called the septa of Underwood. He described different in type, location, size and direction ridges in the MS. According to Underwood, these ridges in the sinus are formed as a result of the development and eruption of teeth, and in the absence of teeth – due to increased osteogenic activity. The septa can be incomplete and complete and divide vertically or horizontally the MS into pockets or cavities. Some of them separate the sinus almost completely and thus chambers are formed with a small drainage communication between them. According to the location of the bony septa, Underwood classified them into three groups: anterior, located between the second premolar and the first molar, middle - between the first and second molar, and posterior - distal to the third molar.

Krennmair et al. [30] analyzed 41 cadaveric maxillary sinuses, 61 sinuses observed during sinus floor augmentation surgeries and 92 computer tomographic scans and reported the frequency, location and height of antral septa in edentulous and non-edentulous patients. The authors found that sinus septa had a higher

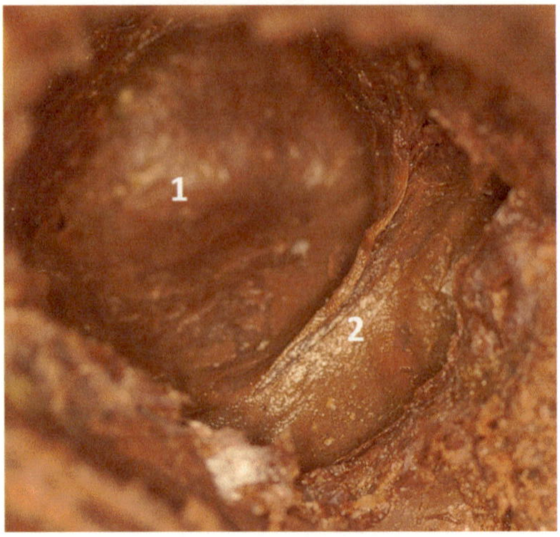

Figure 5.
Septa in the maxillary sinus on cadaveric head: 1 – Maxillary sinus; 2 – Septa.

frequency and lower height in edentulous and atrophic maxillae compared to jaws with preserved dentition. They reported that septa were more common in the anterior regions of the sinus. The authors divided the septa into primary (congenital), which are formed with the normal development of the sinus and the middle facial third [8, 31]; and secondary (acquired), which occur as a result of reshaping of the bone under the action of the masticatory pressure exerted by the teeth. Secondary septa may also occur as a result of tooth loss and bone resorption [29, 31].

The septa are defined as complete when they divide the sinus into separate chambers; and incomplete, dividing the sinus into separate pockets. According to some authors the incidence of the complete septa is 0,3% [32], but it can reach up to 11% [22].

The septa have usually an oblique direction and their function is to absorb and redistribute the masticatory pressure. Occasionally, a bone septum may be found in the sinus, that has formed as a result of the growth of a posterior ethmoid cell in the sinus. It divides it into anterior and posterior compartments. When the septum is horizontal, an upper and lower compartment or a medial and lateral section are separated.

Apart from the floor of the sinus, septa can also arise from its other walls [10, 33], as they are located in two planes – sagittal and transverse. The sagittal septa are most often found in the anterior and middle areas of the sinus, and transverse - in the posterior region [33].

The frequency, location and morphology of septa vary widely.

The frequency of septa varies between 20% and 35% [10, 12, 30]. According to some authors, septa are more common in edentulous alveolar ridges [10, 32], and they are also of greater height.

According to literature, there is no evidence of a relationship between the frequency of bone septa and gender and the age of the individual.

Pommer et al. [32] reported that the incidence of multiple septa in one sinus was 4,2%, and that of bilateral septa was 17,2%.

The distribution of septa in the premolar, molar and retromolar region is 24,4%, 54,6% and 21% respectively [32]. A number of authors reported that the highest incidence of septa is in the middle region [10, 32, 33]. According to other authors, septa are most often located in the posterior area of the sinus [12, 29].

Gosau et al. [12] found that septa are more common in the right sinuses, while according to Pommer et al. [32] their frequency is equal for the left and right sinuses.

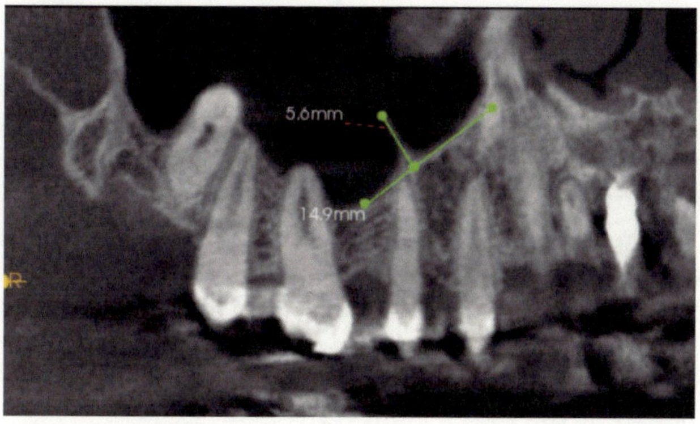

Figure 6.
Height of septa on 3D-cone-beam computer tomography.

According to their shape, the septa can be sagittal, which are most often located in the anterior area of the maxilla; and coronary, which are found in the middle and posterior area of the upper jaw. Coronary septa are divided into three groups: arising from the floor of MS, which are most often transverse; originating from its lateral wall; and septa located in the upper anterior quadrant of the sinus, which are sagittal and are comprised by branches of the infraorbital nerve [10]. Pommer et al. [32] identified three groups of septa - transverse, sagittal and horizontal, with a frequency of 87,6%, 11,1% and 1,3%, respectively.

The average height of septa most often ranges from 5,4 to 7,5 mm [12, 32] (**Figure 6**).

4. Blood supply, lymph drainage and innervation of the maxillary sinus

The blood supply of the MS is mainly by the maxillary artery (MA). It is supplied mainly by three sources: posterior superior alveolar artery (PSAA); infraorbital artery (IOA) and its branches; and lateral posterior nasal arteries - branches of sphenopalatine artery [34]. Arterial blood also comes from the middle nasal concha as the main ostial artery. There are also branches from the anterior and posterior ethmoidal arteries.

The posterior and anterior walls of the sinus are supplied mainly from the posterior superior alveolar and infraorbital arteries.

The PSAA is divided into two branches: an external (gingival branch), which supplies part of the cheek and mucous membrane, covering the alveolar ridge in the area of molars and premolars; and internal (dental branch).

The IOA lies in the infraorbital canal on the inferior orbital wall. In the canal the artery gives off branches for the orbit and the superior anterior alveolar arteries, which supply the gingiva, anterior teeth and premolars, and the corresponding part of the oral mucosa and MS [35].

The gingival branch of PSAA anastomoses with extraosseous branches of the IOA in 10 of 30 sinuses [1]. The dental branch travels anteriorly and inferiorly, passes under the zygomatic process and appears inside the orbit where it also anastomoses with the IOA, forming an arterial circle.

Internal (intraosseous) and external (extraosseous) anastomoses are formed [34, 35]. They supply the Schneiderian membrane, periosteal vestibular tissues and the antero-lateral wall of the sinus [1]. According to the literature data, the incidence of the extraosseous anastomosis ranges from 44–90% [34].

The intraosseous anastomosis is also called alveolar antral artery (AAA) and is of greater clinical importance. It was first described by Strong in 1934. It is most often located in the area where the bone window for sinus lift is prepared. According to various authors and depending on the type of materials used (computer tomography or cadavers), the incidence of AAA varies from 10,5% to 93,9% for computer tomographic studies [36, 37]. In studies on cadavers, the incidence of AAA is 100% [1, 34, 38].

Watanabe et al., 2014 [39] reported that AAA occurs in the area of the first premolar at 28,9%, in the area of the second premolar – in 58,6%, in the area of the first molar – in 48,2%, and in the area of the second molar - in 41,4%.

AAA is entirely intraosseous (in 100% of cases) at its both ends and partially intraosseous in the area from the second premolar to the second molar (in 100% of cases) [1]. Partially the intraosseous part is adjacent to the Schneiderian membrane and is partly enclosed by the lateral sinus wall.

The course of AAA can be intraosseous or intrasinus. The incidence of intraosseous location is higher. According to Kang et al. [40] the intrasinus location was detected in 29,1% of cases. In 26%of the cases the position of the AAA is below the sinus membrane [36]. AAA is located along the outer corticalis of the lateral wall in 5,2–13% of cases [36, 40, 41].

Hur et al. [42] classify the artery as straight (type 1) and U-shaped (type 2). The straight artery occurs much more often (78,1%) compared to U-shaped (21,9%).

According to the literature, the AAA is located at an average distance of 16,4 to 19 mm from the edge of the alveolar ridge [34, 38, 41]. In 20% of cases, it is at a distance of less than 15 mm [38]. Yang et al. [37] found that intraosseous anastomosis is located 19,6 ± 5,64 mm from the edge of the alveolar ridge in the area of the first premolar; 19,9 ± 5,87 mm in the area of the second premolar; at 15,6 ± 4,06 mm in the area of the first molar; and at 16,5 ± 4,75 mm in the area of the second molar. They reported that the distance between the floor of the sinus and the artery is at least at the height of the alveolar ridge of more than 8 mm.

The AAA is found closer to the ridge of the alveolar process (excluding the second molar area) in edentulous patients [43].

The distance between the AAA and the medial sinus wall varies from 11 to 24,9 mm [36, 41].

Extraosseous anastomosis is detected at a distance of 23 to 26 mm [34].

The average length of the intraosseous artery is 44,6 mm and that of the extraosseous is 46 mm [34].

The diameter of the AAA varies from 0,2–3,5 mm, on average 1,09 mm. Arteries with a diameter of less than 1 mm are found in 36,1%, with a diameter between 1 and 2 mm - in 51,4%, and with a diameter of more than 2 mm - in 12,3% [41].

In females, arteries of smaller diameter are found. The diameter of the artery increases with the thickness of the bone wall [40]. In terms of position relative to the upper lateral teeth, the diameter of the AAA slightly decreases to the premolar region [39].

AAA injury is not a life-threatening condition, but it significantly complicates sinus lift operations. The intraosseous artery is of extremely important for determining the length of the dental implant and the position of the incisions in sinus augmentation procedures. Artery injury can cause intense bleeding, difficult visualization of the operative field and subsequently perforation of the Schneiderian membrane. AAA is essential for avoiding local bone necrosis during surgery and for healing the bone graft [38].

The posterior wall of the sinus is supplied by PSAA, greater palatine artery, and branches of the sphenopalatine artery.

The sphenopalatine artery gives off the lateral nasal arteries, which are involved in the blood supply of the maxillary, ethmoid, sphenoidal and frontal sinuses. Branches for the MS enter it through the lateral wall of the nasal cavity.

The venous blood of the sinus is drained by a venous plexus, located around its drainage opening. Anteriorly the venous blood drains into the facial vein and via it – into internal jugular vein; posteriorly – into the maxillary vein, which merges with superficial temporal vein in the parotid gland, forming retromandibular vein, which drains into internal jugular vein. The maxillary vein also anastomoses with the venous pterygoid plexus and via it with the cavernous sinus.

Lymphatic drainage is to a lymphatic plexus, located around the pterygopalatine plexus, to the Eustachian tube and nasopharynx, from where it reaches the lateral cervical and retropharyngeal lymph nodes. Lymphatic vessels from the sinus drain also into the submandibular lymph nodes.

The sensory innervation of the MS is by the maxillary nerve and its branches posterior superior alveolar nerves, middle superior alveolar nerve and anterior superior alveolar nerves, branches of the infraorbital nerve, posterior inferior nasal branches (greater palatine nerve). The ostium of the sinus is innervated by the greater palatine nerve. The glands located in the mucosa of the MS receive post-ganglionar parasympathetic fibers from the greater petrosal nerve, a branch of *n. intermedius* of the facial nerve. The vasoconstrictor innervation is by means of sympathetic fibers, originating from the carotid plexus.

5. Histology of the maxillary sinus

The walls of the MS are covered with a mucous membrane, which is made up of epithelium (lamina epithelialis), lying on a basement membrane, and subepithelial connective tissue (lamina propria). The mucous membrane of the sinus is thinner than that of the nasal cavity, contains fewer blood vessels and is therefore pale blue in color. In the MS its thickness is approximately about 0,3–0,8 mm [44]. However, in smokers it varies widely, and the epithelium is usually squamous.

The epithelium is pseudostratified columnar ciliated epithelium. It originates from the respiratory epithelium of the nasal mucosa. In addition to the typical columnar ciliated cells, there are also basal (stem) cells, columnar cells without cilia and goblet cells that produce and secrete mucin.

The cilated cells have an electronic-light cytoplasm in which a large number of mitochondria, organelles producing enzymes and basal bodies are detected. The basal bodies play the role of attaching apparatus for cylindrical microtubules to the cell membrane in the apical part of the cell. The cilia are approximately 50–200 in number and are composed of 9 + 1 pairs of microtubules. The rate of their oscillations, which are synchronous and undulating, is 700–800 beats/minute [45]. The motor activity of the cilia is not regulated in a nervous way but is automatic. They help to purify the sinus epithelium from the debris, microorganisms and mucus secretion that move in the direction of the ostium and through it to the nasal cavity. Due to the high location of the drainage opening, the ciliated cells must overcome gravity. The speed of movement of secretions is 9 mm/sec [45].

The non-ciliated columnar cells possess microvili, which significantly increase the surface of the epithelium, which helps to better warm and moisturize the air.

Basal cells are inherently stem cells that give the beginning of different types of epithelial cells.

The goblet cells are single-celled glands that synthesize and secrete mucus. In their shape, they resemble inverted wine glasses. The nucleus is located at their basal end, and secretory granules - at their apical end. They produce glycoproteins and thus increase the viscosity and elasticity of the mucus secretion produced by the subepithelial glands. The goblet cells pour their secretion by merging the secretory granules with their cell membrane with its subsequent rupture. Therefore, these cells are apocrine. They are in the largest amount in the MS - 9600 mm^2 [44].

Lamina propria is much thinner compared to this of the mucosa of the nasal cavity. It is composed mainly of loose connective tissue. In the intercellular space are found mainly collagen and a small number of elastic fibers. This layer is moderately blood supplied and contains subepithelial antral glands. These glands are of a mixed nature and are composed of serous and mucus acini or sero-mucus acini and myoepithelial cells. The antral glands are in a particularly large amount around the drainage opening of the sinus. They secrete their secretions through their excretory ducts. When stimulated by the parasympathetic system, they secrete a thick mucus secretion, and when stimulated by the sympathetic system, the secretion is sparse.

On the surface of the mucous membrane, a mucous covering is formed, which is composed of two layers. The first is a *sol* layer *(serous layer).* It is thin, produced by the microvilli and facilitates the movements of the cilia. It serves as a lubricant. The second is a *gel* layer *(surface mucoid layer)*. It is located on the surface of the mucosa and is a thick mucus secretion, composed mainly of glycoproteins. This secretion is produced by the goblet cells and subepithelial glands. Thanks to it, the underlying mucous membrane is protected from low temperatures and humidity. The secretion also has a cleansing function, as it captures foreign particles and microorganisms. It also contains factors of the immune system: Ig A, Ig G and interferon, lactoferrin, lysozyme.

In the healthy sinus there is a continuous cycle, which consists in the production of mucus secretion, its movement through the cilia of epithelial cells and drainage through the ostium. Serous and goblet cells produce up to 1 l. secretion per day. The cilia of epithelial cells and the produced secretion form the muco-ciliary transport system. Muco-ciliary clearance is responsible for the continuous removal of foreign substances on the mucous membrane.

Bacterial or viral infections, contaminants, allergens, smoking negatively affect the normal activity of the ciliated epithelium. The functioning of the muco-ciliary transport depends to a large extent on the patency of the drainage opening and on the adequate supply of oxygen to the sinus. Obstruction of the drainage opening is due to edema of the nasal mucosa, which leads to the retention of secretion in the sinus, to the resorption of gases and the creation of negative pressure, which facilitates the invasion of pathogenic microorganisms. On the other hand, when the sinus ostium is permeable, the environment in the sinus is aerobic and normal ciliary function is present. When the opening is impermeable, the environment becomes anaerobic, and as a result, the bacterial flora in the sinus changes. The colonization and growth of anaerobic bacteria, which cause the development of maxillary sinusitis, is favored.

With inflammation of the mucosa, there is a sharp reduction to complete paralysis of the movements of the cilia under the influence of toxins of viruses and bacteria, as a result of which their cleansing effect is affected. In chronic rhinosinusitis, limited or diffuse epithelial metaplasia and impaired transport function may occur. As a result, there are edema of the mucous membrane, accumulation of mucus secretion and bacterial colonization.

The sinus mucosa is firmly attached to the underlying periosteum, which is why it is referred to as a muco-periosteal membrane. This membrane is called Schneiderian. The muco-periosteum is loosely attached to the underlying bone, therefore peels off easily. It contains osteoclasts and osteoblasts. The thickness of the Schneiderian membrane can vary widely – 0,16–34,61 mm [46].

Very often as a result of various pathological processes the Schneiderian membrane thickens, which further complicates the treatment of rhinosinusitis and sinus augmentation surgery. Therefore, the assessment of the thickness of the sinus mucosa is of great importance for endoscopic sino-nasal surgery and oral implantology. Mucosal thickness higher than 2 mm is considered pathological [46]. Odontogenic sinusitis develops as a result of chronic limited inflammation, a cyst or granuloma at the root of the upper premolars and molars, or as a result of foreign body or root filling during tooth extraction and endodontic treatment. There is a direct relationship between the presence of periapical processes and the thickness of the Schneider membrane. The thickening of the sinus mucosa increases proportionally with the degree of apical periodontitis. By lesions infiltrating the floor of the MS, pathological mucosal thickening occurs in 90% [47]. The thickness of the Schneiderian membrane is greater near restored teeth and periodontal and endodontic lesions, and this dependence is strongly expressed in the molar areas, when there is a thin bone plate between the dental roots and sinus or periapical lesions are present [47, 48]. Other factors for mucosal thickening are infections, allergies, smoking.

The frequency of thickening of the sinus mucosa varies widely - from 34–66% [47, 48]. The frequency of thickening of the Schneiderian membrane increases with age, and it is highest in the age group 40–60 years. With roots, protruding into the sinus, a higher incidence of mucosal thickening is also observed.

Most often, the thickness of the mucous membrane is 2–4 mm, its average is 2,70 ± 3,73 mm [47]. According to Bozhikova et al. [48] the Schneiderian membrane thickness ranged between 0 and 15,90 mm, average 2,24 ± 3,11 mm. The highest mean values (2,16 – 3,11 mm) were found in the middle sagittal region of the MS. In the presence of sinusitis, the average thickening of the membrane reaches 7.4 mm [49]. Flat thickening of the Schneiderian membrane is most common [46].

6. Physiology of the sinuses

There is still no consensus on the functions of paranasal sinuses. It is assumed that they help moisturize and warm the inhaled air; provide voice resonance; increase the olfactory surface; regulate intranasal pressure; their mucosa secretes mucin, which further moisturizes the nasal cavity; promote facial growth; reduce the mass of the skull; build a kind of framework for the brain and absorb the shock effects of injuries to the face and skull, reducing their severity.

The mucous membranes of the nasal cavities and sinuses form a single transport system that protects the respiratory tract. In the sinuses, the secretions move only to their drainage openings. The muco-ciliary system captures 80% of inhaled solid particles between 3 and 5 micrometers in size and 60% of particles more than 2 micrometers in size. These particles are exposed to the action of mast cells, polymorphonuclear leukocytes, eosinophils, lysozyme, immunoglobulins and interferon.

7. Conclusion

Preliminary assessment of the morphology of the MS – linear dimensions and volume, bone wall thickness, presence of septa, locations and permeability of the maxillary ostium, thickness of the sinus mucosa, relations to the neighboring structures are prerequisite for diagnosis and treatment of sinus diseases, and restoration of the edentulous distal maxilla. The study of the sinus anatomy allows to determine its degree of pneumatization, the position of its ostium, the thickness of the mucosa, to detect the anatomical variations and to diagnose the pathological process in it. These parameters are essential when conducting various dental, nasal and paranasal procedures, as in many cases may complicate or compromise treatment. Conducting sino-nasal surgery and implant treatment of the distal area of the maxilla is impossible without assessment of the morphology of the sinus in order to prepare an appropriate treatment plan, prevention of intra- and postoperative complications and prediction of the results of treatment.

Author details

Elena Bozhikova[1*] and Nikolay Uzunov[2]

1 Department of Anatomy, Histology and Embryology, Faculty of Medicine, Medical University, Plovdiv, Bulgaria

2 Private Practice, Plovdiv, Bulgaria

*Address all correspondence to: elibozhikova@gmail.com

References

[1] Rosano G, Taschieri S, Gaudy JF, Del Fabbro M. Maxillary sinus vascularization: a cadaveric study. J Craniofac Surg, 2009;20(3):940-943. DOI: 10.1097/SCS.0b013e3181a2d77f

[2] Farah G, Nafis AF. Morphometric analysis of developing maxillary sinuses in human foetuses. Int. J. Morphol, 2006;24(3):303-308.

[3] Nuñez-Castruita A, Lopez-Serna N, Guzman-Lopez S. Prenatal development of the maxillary sinus: a perspective for paranasal sinus surgery. Otolaryngol Head Neck Surg, 2012;146(6):997-1003. DOI: 10.1177/0194599811435883

[4] Barghouth G, Prior JO, Lepori D, Duvoisin B, Schnyder P, Gudinchet F. Paranasal sinuses in children: size evaluation of maxillary, sphenoid and frontal sinuses by magnetic resonance imaging and proposal of volume index percentile curves. Eur Radiol, 2002;12(6):1451-1458. DOI: 10.1007/s00330-001-1218-9

[5] Proetz A. Essays on the Applied Physiology of the Nose. St. Louis: Annals Publishing, 1953

[6] Alberti P. Applied surgical anatomy of the maxillary sinus. Otolaryngol Clin North Am, 1976;9:3-20. DOI: 10.1016/S0030-6665(20)32713-4

[7] Bozhikova E, Uzunov N, Kitova T, Iotova N. Morphometric study of maxillary sinus on cadavers. USB, 2019;23:310-314.

[8] Chanavaz M. Maxillary sinus: anatomy, physiology, surgery, and bone grafting related to implantology - eleven years of surgical experience (1979-1990). J Oral Implantol, 1990;16(3): 199-209.

[9] Stammberger H. Functional endoscopic sinus surgery. The Messerklinger technique. Philadelphia: BC Decker, 1990;247:63-76.

[10] Ghandi KR, Wabale RN, Siddiqui AU. The incidence and morphology of maxillary sinus septa in dentate and edentulous maxillae: a cadaveric study with a brief review of the literature. J Korean Assoc Oral Maxilofac Surg, 2015;41(1):30-36. DOI: 10.5125/jkaoms.2015.41.1.30

[11] De Haven HA. Clinical Maxillary Sinus Elevation Surgery. 1st ed. John Wiley & Sons Inc Publ; 2014.

[12] Gosau M, Rink D, Driemel O, Draeurt FG. Maxillary sinus anatomy: A cadaveric study with clinical implication. Anat Rec (Hoboken), 2009;292(3):352- 354. DOI: 10.1002/ar.20859

[13] Kumar RH, Kaka RS. Accessory maxillary ostia: topography and clinical application. J Anat Soc India, 2001;50:3-5

[14] Jones NS. CT of the paranasal sinuses: A review of the correlation with clinical, surgical and histopathological findings. Clin Otolaryngol Allied Sci, 2002;27:11-17. DOI: 10.1046/j.0307-7772.2001.00525.x

[15] Matthews BL, Burke AJ. Recirculation of mucus via accessory ostia causing chronic maxillary sinus disease. Otolaryngol Head Neck Surg, 1997;117:422-423. DOI: 10.1016/S0194-5998(97)70139-6

[16] Monje A, Catena A, Monje F, Gonzalez-Garsia R, Galindo-Moreno P, Suarez F, et al. Maxillary sinus lateral wall thickness and morphologic patterns in the atrophic posterior maxilla. J Periodontol, 2014;85(5):676-682. DOI: 10.1902/jop.2013.130392

[17] Yang SM, Park SI, Kye SB, Shin SY. Computed tomographic assessment of

maxillary sinus wall thickness in edentulous patients. J Oral Rehabil, 2012;39:421-428. DOI: 10.1111/ j.1365-2842.2012.02295.x

[18] Monje A, Monje F, Gonzales-Garcia R, Suarez F, Galindo-Moreno P, Garcia-Nogales A, et al. Influence of atrophic posterior maxilla ridge height on bone density and microarchitecture. Clin Implant Dent Relat Res, 2015;17(1):111- 119. DOI: 10.1111/cid.12075

[19] Hamdy RM, Abdel-Wahed N. Three-dimensional linear and volumetric analysis of maxillary sinus pneumatization. J Ady Res, 2014;5:387-395. DOI: 10.1016/j.jare.2013.06.006

[20] Nimigean V, Nimigean VR, Maru N, Sălăvăstru DI, Bădită D, Tuculină MJ. The maxillary sinus floor in the oral implantology. Rom J Morphol Embryol, 2008;49(4):485-489.

[21] Mattar E, Hammad L, Faden A, Khalil H. Relation of maxillary teeth to the maxillary sinus in normal Saudi individuals living in Riyadh. Biosci Biotech Res Asia, 2010;7(2):695-700.

[22] Bozhikova E. Morphological aspects of the maxillary sinus [thesis]. Plovdiv: Medical University of Plovdiv; 2020.

[23] Kilic C, Kamburoglu K, Yuksel SP, Ozen T. An assessment of the relationship between the maxillary sinus floor and the maxillary posterior teeth root tips using dental cone-beam computerized tomography. Eur J Dent, 2010;4:462-467.

[24] Shokri A, Lari S, Yousef F, Hashemi L. Assessment of the relationship between the maxillary sinus floor and maxillary posterior teeth roots using cone beam computed tomography. J Contemp Dent Pract, 2014;15(5):618-622. DOI: 10.5005/ jp-journals-10024-1589

[25] Freisfeld M, Drescher D, Schellmann B, Schüller H. The maxillary sixth-year molar and its relation to the maxillary sinus. A comparative study between the panoramic tomogram and the computed tomogram. Fortschritte der Kieferorthop, 1993;54(5):179-186. DOI: 10.1007/BF02341464

[26] Kwak HH, Park HD, Yoon HR, Kang MK, Koh KS, Kim HJ. Topographic anatomy of the inferior wall of the maxillary sinus in Koreans. Int J Oral Maxillofac Surg, 2004;33:382-388. DOI: 10.1016/j.ijom.2003.10.012

[27] Didilescu A, Rusu M, Săndulescu M, Georgescu C, Ciuluyică. Morphometric analysis of the relationships between the maxillary first molar and maxillary sinus floor. OJST, 2012;2:352-357. DOI: 10.4236/ojst.2012.24060

[28] Underwood A.S. Surgical considerations connected with the anatomy of the maxillary sinus. Br Med J, 1909;15:1. DOI: 10.1136/ bmj.1.2524.1178

[29] Underwood A. S. An inquiry into the anatomy and pathology of the maxillary sinus. J Anat Physiol, 1910;44(Pt 4):354-369.

[30] Krennmair G, Ulm CW, Lugmayr H, Solar P. The incidence, location, and height of maxillary sinus septa in the edentulousand dentate maxilla. Int J Oral Max Surg, 1999;57:667-671. DOI: 10.1016/s0278-2391(99)90427-5

[31] Ulm CW, Solar P, Gsellmann B, Matejka M, Watzek G. The edentulous maxillary alveolar process in the region of the maxillary sinus - a study of physical dimension. Int J Oral Maxillofac Surg, 1995;24(4):279-282. DOI: 10.1016/s0901-5027(95)80029-8

[32] Pommer B, Ulm C, Lorenzoni M, Palmer R, Watzek G, Zechner W. Prevalence, location and morphology of

maxillary sinus septa: systematic review and meta-analysis. J Clin Periodontol, 2012;39:769-773. DOI: 10.1111/j1600-051X.2012.01897.x

[33] Rosano G, Taschieri S, Gaudy JF, Lesmes D, Del Fabbro M. Maxillary sinus septa: a cadaveric study. J Oral Maxillofac Surg, 2010;68:1360-1364. DOI: 10.1016/j.joms.2009.07069

[34] Solar P, Geyerhofer U, Traxler H, Windisch A, Ulm C, Watzek G. Blood supply to the maxillary sinus relevant to sinus elevation procedures. Clin Oral Implants Res, 1999;10:34-44. DOI: 10.1034/j.1600-0501.1999.100105.x

[35] Flanagan D. Arterial supply of maxillary sinus and potential for bleeding complication during lateral approach sinus elevation. Implant Dent, 2005;14:336-338. DOI: 10.1097/01.id.0000188437.66363.7c

[36] Shahidi S, Zamiri B, Danaei SM, Selehi s, Hamedani S. Evaluation of anatomic variations in maxillary sinus with the aid of cone beam computed tomography (CBCT) in a population in South of Iran. J Dent Shiraz UnivMed Sci, 2016;17(1):7-15.

[37] Yang SM, Kye SB. Location of maxillary intraosseous vascular anastomosis based on the tooth position and height of the residual alveolar bone: computed tomographic analysis. J Periodontal implant Sci, 2014;44(2):50-56. DOI: 10.5051/jpis.2014.44.2.50

[38] Traxler H, Windisch A, Geyerhofer U, Surd R, Solar P, Firbas W. Arterial blood supply of the maxillary sinus. Clin Anat, 1999;12:417-421. DOI: 10.1002/ (SICI)1098-2353(1999)12:63.0.CO;2-W

[39] Watanabe T, Shiota M, Gao S, Imakita C, Tachikawa N, Kasugas S. Verification of posterior superior alveolar artery distribution in lateral wall of maxillary sinus by location and defect pattern. Quintessence Int, 2014;45:673-678. DOI: 10.3290/j.qi.a32239

[40] Kang SJ, Shin SI, Herr Y, Kwon Y Kim G, Chung J. Anatomical structures in the maxillary sinus related to latera; sinus elevation; a cone-beam computed tomographic analysis. Clin oral Implants Res, 2013;24:75-81. DOI: 10.1111/j.1600-0501.2011.02378.x

[41] Güncü GN, Yildirim YD, Wang HL, Tözüm TF. Location of posterior superior alveolar artery and evaluation of maxillary sinus anatomy with computerized tomography: a clinical study. Clin Oral Implants Res, 2011;22:1164-1167. DOI: 10.1111/j.1600-0501.2010.02071.x

[42] Hur MS, Kim JK, Hu KS, Bae Kyong HE, Park H, Kim H. Clinical implications of the topography and distribution of the posterior superior alveolar artery. J Craniofac Surg, 2009;20(2):551-554. DOI: 10.1097/CSC.0b013e31819ba1c1

[43] Park WH, Choi SY, Kim CS. Study on the position of the posterior superior alveolar artery in relation to the performance of the maxillary sinus bone graft procedure in a Korean population. J Korean Assoc Oral Maxillofac Surg, 2012;38:71-77. DOI: 10.5125/jkaoms.2012.38.2.71

[44] Morgensen C. Quantitative histology of the maxillary sinus. Rhinology, 1977;15(3):129-140.

[45] Watelet JB, Van Cauwenberge P. Applied anatomy and physiology of the nose and paranasal sinuses. Allergy 1999;54:14-25. DOI: 10.1111/j.1398-9995.1999.tb04402.x

[46] Janner SF, Caversaccio MD, Dubach P, Sendi P, Buser D, Bornstein M. Characteristics and

dimensions of the Schneiderian membrane: a radiographic analysis using cone beam computed tomography in patients referred for dental implant surgery in the posterior maxilla. Clin Oral Implants Res, 2011;22:1446-1453. DOI: 10.1111/j.1600-0501.2010.021140.x

[47] Goller-Bulut D, Sekerci A, Köse E, Sisman Y. Cone beam computed tomographic analysis of maxillary premolars and molars to detect the relationship between periapical and marginal bone loss and mucosal thickness of maxillary sinus. Med Oral Patol Oral Cir Bucal, 2015;20(5):e572-579. DOI: 10.4317/medoral.20587

[48] Bozhikova E, Uzunov N, Kitova T. Cone-beam computed tomographic study of mucosal thickness of maxillary sinus floor. Acta Morphologica et Anthropologica, 2019; 26(3-4):116-125.

[49] Maillet M, Bowles WR, McClanahan SL, John MT, Ahmad M. Cone-beam computed tomography evaluation of maxillary sinusitis. J Endodontics, 2011;37(6):753-757. DOI: 10.1016/j.joen.2011.02.032

Chapter 2

Infectious Causes of Acute and Chronic Sinusitis

Jana I. Preis, Anna W. Maro, Sophie Hurez and Sneha Pusapati

Abstract

Paranasal sinuses anatomy is paired in 4 parts which includes frontal, maxillary, ethmoid, and sphenoid. Their relevant function is to secrete mucous for moisture, humidify inspired air, impart vocal resonance, and act as shock absorber for intracranial contents. Retention of secretions in the nasal cavity and sinuses can cause inflammation of the mucosa of paranasal sinuses and lead to infection. Classification of sinusitis is based on duration of symptoms. Diagnosis can be achieved clinically, however other diagnosis modalities such as cultures or radiology can help to achieve accurate diagnosis. Depending on the etiology management can be supportive or pharmacological. In some cases, long term monitoring and prevention therapy may be required.

Keywords: Sinusitis, rhinosinusitis

1. Introduction

Sinusitis is the inflammation of the mucosa of Paranasal sinuses (frontal, ethmoidal, sphenoid, maxillary sinuses). Rhinitis is the inflammation of the mucosal membranes of the nose. Rhino sinusitis refers to the inflammation of the mucosal membranes of the nose and at least one of the Paranasal sinuses. Sinusitis is almost always preceded by rhinitis and often occurs together. Hence rhinosinusitis and sinusitis are often used interchangeably.

Rhinosinusitis is one of the 10 most common conditions seen by primary care physicians. The prevalence of Acute rhinosinusitis (ARS) varies between 6 and 15%. The prevalence of chronic sinusitis is 12.5%. Yearly incidence: sinusitis affects 1 in 7 adults and is diagnosed in 31 million patients. Acute bacterial infection occurs in only 0.5 to 2.0 percent of episodes of ARS. The incidence is higher in women and among those aged 45 to 64 years. The direct costs of sinusitis, including medications, outpatient and emergency department visits, and ancillary tests and procedures, are estimated to be $3 billion per year in the United States. Rhinosinusitis is the fifth most common diagnosis for which antibiotics are prescribed. It causes a wide array of symptoms, negatively affects quality of life, and can cause significant impairment in daily functioning.

2. Risk factors

Rhinosinusitis often occurs in the early spring (often associated with upper respiratory tract infection which occurs in colder months). The incidence of URTI is itself extensive, averages to 2–3 episodes in adults and 6–8 episodes in children. 0.5% of patients proceed to rhinosinusitis. Ventilation disorders of the sinuses can also lead to sinusitis; nasal polyps, deviated nasal septum, cystic fibrosis, primary ciliary dyskinesia, or granulomatosis with polyangiitis- odontogenic infections, bronchial asthma, and analgesic (NSAIDs, aspirin) intolerance. Foreign bodies caught in the nasal cavity, particularly seen in children, also puts them at risk for rhinosinusitis. Other important risk factors for the development of sinusitis, include age as described above, female gender, smoking, and immunodeficiency, air travel, exposure to changes in atmospheric pressure (eg, deep sea diving), swimming, and even anxiety and depression.

3. Classification

Sinusitis is classified based on duration of symptoms (**Table 1**). Acute rhinosinusitis (ARS) as mentioned lasts less than 4 weeks in duration. Underlying etiology is most often viral from URTI and less commonly bacterial. The challenge in treating ARS is based on the physician's ability to distinguish the etiology between bacterial and viral and determine if the patient will benefit from antibiotics. Bacterial and prolonged viral illnesses have similar presentations, complicating the assessment. Majority of patients with viral sinusitis have a complete recovery in a week. Even in patients with bacterial etiology, $2/3^{rd}$recover without any antibiotic therapy although the duration of symptoms may be prolonged. Based on the underlying etiology ARS can be further classified based on the etiology and complications.

1. Acute viral rhinosinusitis (AVRS) – ARS with viral etiology.

2. Uncomplicated acute bacterial rhinosinusitis (ABRS) – ARS with bacterial etiology without clinical evidence of extension outside the paranasal sinuses and nasal cavity (e.g., without neurologic, ophthalmologic, or soft tissue involvement).

3. Complicated ABRS – ARS with bacterial etiology with clinical evidence of extension outside the paranasal sinuses and nasal cavity.

The most common viral pathogens are rhinovirus, coronavirus, adenovirus, influenza, and parainfluenza virus. Other less common pathogens causing this disease are bacteria. The most common community acquired bacterial organisms are *Streptococcus Pneumoniae* and Haemophilus influenza, both accounting for 75% of cases. On the other hand, nosocomial infections are associated with gram-negative organisms, noted in prolonged intubation. Dental procedures and infections are associated with anaerobic and microaerophilic bacteria. Fungal infections are

Classification	Duration of symptoms
Acute	Up to 4 weeks
Subacute	At least four weeks but less than twelve weeks
Recurrent	Four or more episodes per year with complete resolution between episodes; each episode lasts at least seven days
Chronic	12 weeks or longer

Table 1.
Showing classification of sinusitis based on duration of symptoms [1].

seen in immunocompromised individuals, often caused by aspergillus and Mucor. *Staphylococcus aureus*, *Moraxella catarrhalis* and gram-negative organisms which predominate in chronic rhinosinusitis.

4. Anatomy and pathophysiology

There are 4 paired paranasal sinuses (frontal, maxillary, ethmoid, and sphenoid). The sinuses impart various functions. Relevant functions include imparting vocal resonance, filter, and humidify inspired air, warm the inspired air, act as shock absorbers for intracranial contents, and secrete mucus for moisture. The mucosal lining of the sinuses is pseudostratified ciliated columnar epithelium. Below the epithelium lies the basement membrane, below that is the lamina propria with lymphoid tissue and secretory glands. Goblet cells are also present interspersed with the epithelial cells.

The ostium of the maxillary sinus drains into the middle meatus in the hiatus semilunaris. Accessory ostia can be present in 25–30% of the population. Anterior ethmoid cells also drain into the hiatus semilunaris through the infundibulum. Posterior ethmoid cells drain through the superior meatus. The frontal sinus drains via the nasofrontal duct into the infundibulum of the middle meatus. The sphenoid sinus opens into the sphenoethmoid recess above the superior concha (**Figure 1**).

The primary pathogenesis that leads to infection is retention of secretions in the nasal cavity and the sinuses. There are various defense mechanisms in place. The mucous blanket which travels at 1 cm/min traps and propels any irritants towards the nasopharynx with the help of cilia, together known as the mucociliary system. Around 1liter per day of mucus is produced. Secretory IgA is also present to protect against pathogens. The breakdown of these defense systems is followed by retention of secretions. Various factors impeding the mucociliary system include mucosal swelling with closing of ostia, ciliary abnormalities, and overproduction of the secretions. The disruption of the mucociliary system and retention of secretions results in closing of the draining ostia, especially maxillary and sphenoid sinuses which drain upwards against gravity. As the ostial size reduces, the movement of air is reduced, and oxygen tensions drop. Along with that, the carbon dioxide levels increase, and pH is lowered. All these conditions favor further pathogen growth. The pathogens produce a vicious cycle as they further cause ciliary dyskinesia and thickened secretions.

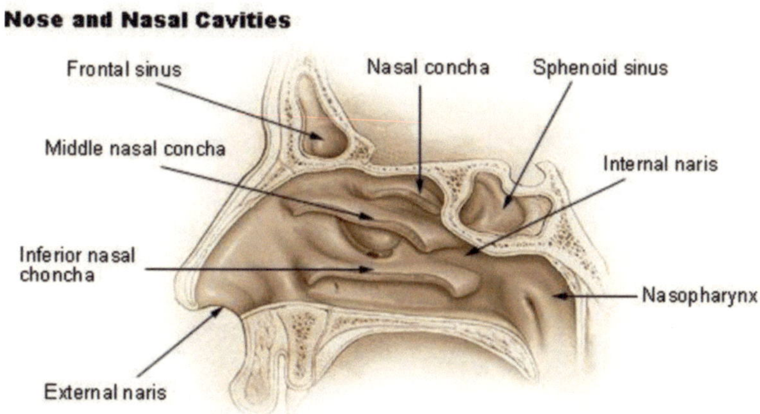

Figure 1.
Showing the anatomy of nose and nasal cavities. Image courtesy of [2, 3].

Acute viral rhinosinusitis (AVR) is transmitted by direct contact with conjunctival or nasal mucosa and viral levels can be detected within 10 hours and symptoms often develop within one day in a non-immune individual. Acute bacterial rhinosinusitis (ABRS) occurs in 0.5–2% of all ARS due to secondary infection of the already inflamed cavity by a viral infection. It can also be associated with any other condition impairing the defense mechanism mentioned above. ABRS is often caused by high concentration of a single pathogens but noted to be two pathogens in approximately 25% of the patients.

5. Clinical presentation

5.1 Symptoms

ARS symptoms include (a) nasal congestion or obstruction (b) purulent nasal discharge (c) maxillary tooth discomfort (d) facial pain or pressure that is worse or localized to sinuses when bending forward. Various other possible symptoms are listed below. Note the symptoms associated with middle ear infection and eustachian tube dysfunction (**Table 2**).

Purulent discharge must be present for the diagnosis of acute rhinosinusitis. Purulent discharge is cloudy or colored which is not seen in the case of an upper respiratory tract infection (clear discharge-rhinorrhea). It is a helpful distinction.

The facial pain or pressure most commonly involves the maxillary sinuses- over the cheeks- and often mimics dental pain. Other sinuses involved are the frontal sinuses-lower forehead- ethmoidal sinuses-nasal bridge and/or between the eyes or retro-orbital pain and sphenoid sinus- near sphenoid bones, most posterior sinuses.

Distinguishing AVRS from ABRS as we discussed is essential and relies on the clinical course of the conditions (**Table 3**). Only 50% of cases are accurately diagnosed with bacterial sinusitis. In ABRS, symptoms often persist beyond 10 days with failure to improve. Or there are at least 3 initial days of severe symptoms, fever (> 39°or 102°F), facial pain, or purulent nasal discharge. Or the symptoms initially improve and then worsen after 5–6 days (double worsening). In AVRS, symptoms often improve by day 10 although may persist for days after. Fever may be present but often disappears within 24–48 hours with respiratory symptoms becoming more prominent after. Purulent discharge is a sign of inflammation and cannot be used to distinguish between the two.

Symptoms of acute rhinosinusitis
Purulent nasal discharge
Facial fullness or congestion
Nasal congestion or obstruction
Hyposmia or anosmia
Fever
Headache
Ear pain, pressure, or fullness
Halitosis
Dental pain
Fatigue

Table 2.
Showing symptoms of acute rhinosinusitis.

Term	Definition
Acute rhinosinusitis (ARS)	Lasting up to 4 weeks of purulent nasal discharge with associated nasal obstruction, facial pain/pressure/fullness, or both. Cloudy or colored purulent nasal discharge, as oppose to clear secretions that typically seen in upper respiratory viral infection, may be reported, or seen on physical examination. Facial pain-pressure-fullness may manifest as diffuse or localized headache and may involve anterior face or periorbital region
Viral rhinosinusitis (VRS)	Acute rhinosinusitis that is caused by viral infection, usually diagnosed when signs and symptoms of acute rhinosinusitis are present less than 10 days and not worsening
Acute bacterial rhinosinusitis (ABRS)	signs or symptoms of acute rhinosinusitis fail to improve within 10 days or more beyond the onset of upper respiratory symptoms, or Signs or symptoms of acute rhinosinusitis worsen within 10 days after initial

Table 3.
Distinguishing between ASR, VRS and ABRS based on signs and symptoms.

The below diagram is a helpful guide to distinguish between the various phenotypes (**Figure 2**).

Chronic rhinosinusitis (CRS) may present acutely without improvement of symptoms or insidiously over months to years. Must be present for at least 12 weeks with at least two of the following symptoms: mucopurulent drainage, nasal congestion (obstruction), facial pain-pressure-fullness, anosmia or hyposmia. Following signs of inflammation must also be present with 1 or more findings such as purulent mucus or edema in the middle meatus/anterior ethmoidal area during anterior rhinoscopy, polyps in the nasal cavity/middle meatus and imaging showing inflammation of the paranasal sinuses. Additional symptoms of CRS may include halitosis, dental pain, or other non-specific features. Therefore, the differential diagnosis of CRS is broad and includes allergic rhinitis, nonallergic rhinitis, vasomotor rhinitis, eosinophilic nonallergic rhinitis or nasal septal deformity. CRS is further divided between CRS with nasal polyps and CRS without nasal polyps.

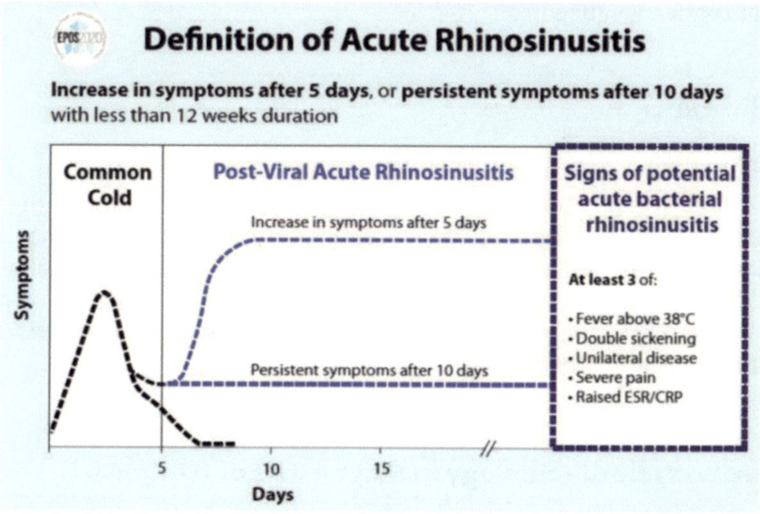

Figure 2.
Duration of symptoms to differentiate ARS (common cold) which is 5 days and Post-viral ARS which is longer than 10 days. Bacterial ARS should be suspected in presence of 3 or more symptoms [4].

Term	Definition
Chronic rhinosinusitis	Twelve weeks or longer of two or more of the following symptoms • Mucopurulent drainage (posterior, anterior, or both) • Nasal congestion or obstruction • Facial pain-pressure-fullness, or • Decrease sense of smell PLUS, Inflammation documented by one or more of the following findings: • Purulent mucous or edema in the middle meatus, and or • Radiographic evidence for inflammation of the paranasal sinuses
Recurrent acute rhinosinusitis	Four or more episodes per year of acute bacterial rhinosinusitis (ABRS) without signs or symptoms of rhinosinusitis between episodes

Table 4.
Distinguishing between chronic rhinosinusitis and recurrent acute rhinosinusitis.

Recurrent acute rhinosinusitis presents with 4 or more episodes per year of ABRS without signs or symptoms of rhinosinusitis between episodes. Each episode lasts at least 7 days (**Table 4**).

6. Physical findings

Signs of ARS include cardinal signs of inflammation. Erythema and edema may be seen over the cheek bones or periorbital area. Tenderness may be present at the site of the sinuses which aggravates with percussion. Transillumination, which is the process of using a bright light applied to the skin over a lesion to assess for transmission of light, can be used over the maxillary or frontal sinuses. In the case of rhinosinusitis, it may show opacification. Both percussion and transillumination have low sensitivity and specificity and are not useful in making a diagnosis. Anterior rhinoscopy examination using an otoscope may show swelling and hypertrophy of the turbinate and reflex narrowing of the meatus. Purulent discharge may be noted. Anatomic abnormalities such as polyps or septal deviation may be visualized.

7. Complications

Although rare, complications of ARBS can include pre septal cellulitis, orbital cellulitis, subperiosteal abscess, osteomyelitis of the sinus bones, meningitis, intracranial abscess, and septic cavernous sinus thrombosis. Symptoms that should prompt immediate evaluation include severe and persistent headache, periorbital inflammation, vision changes, proptosis or abnormal extraocular movements, cranial nerve palsies, AMS, signs of meningitis or any signs of increased intracranial pressure.

8. Diagnostics/role of radiology in diagnostics of ID sinusitis

The diagnosis of acute rhinosinusitis (ARS) is achieved clinically. Getting adequate sinus cultures from sinus aspiration ($\geq 10^4$ colony-forming units per milliliter, non-contaminated) remains problematic. In addition, sinus aspiration is invasive and time-consuming. Diagnosing ARS relies first on ruling out upper respiratory tract infection (URTI), then accurately distinguishing ABRS from AVRS.

ARS differentiates itself from URTI based on signs and symptoms with the former presenting with purulent nasal drainage accompanied by nasal obstruction, facial pain-pressure-fullness, or both. URTI lacks such features and instead will present with features of rhinitis (sneezing, post-nasal drip, rhinorrhea) and pharyngitis (sore throat, cough). Such features are often present in ARS.

Once ARS has been clinically diagnosed, the etiology of ARS must be characterized, and this is done by looking at the temporal pattern and the severity of the illness. ABRS persists beyond 10 days and there is failure to improve in 10 days. Double worsening may also be seen where the symptoms initially improve and then worsen after 5–6 days. In AVRS, symptoms are present for less than 10 days and symptoms are not worsening.

Imaging and endoscopy are not indicated for diagnosis of ARS and cannot be used to distinguish ABRS from AVRS. They are only indicated when there are suspected complications such as red flag symptoms (focal neurological deficits, severe headache, facial numbness, proptosis, blurry vision, swelling, impaired ocular movements, symptoms not improving despite adequate antibiotics therapy). Imaging and endoscopy are also indicated when risk factors for invasive fungal rhinitis are present (immunocompromised, diabetes mellitus) or in the case of recurrent ARS or CRS. In CRS, presence of inflammation seen in anterior rhinoscopy, nasal endoscopy or sinus CT is needed for diagnosis.

When imaging is indicated, sinus computed tomography (CT) is the gold standard. Sinus X-ray is no longer recommended due to low sensitivity and specificity. Sinus CT helps quantify the extent of inflammation, identify polyps or anatomical abnormalities, and rule out neoplasm or severe fungal infections. Sinus CT is required if endoscopic sinus surgery is planned.

When red flag symptoms are present, CT with contrast is preferred whereas CT without contrast is sufficient for recurrent ABRS and CRS. Findings of ARS on sinus CT are non-specific (opacification, mucosal thickening, air-fluid levels, soft tissue swelling). In CRS, sinus CT may show etiology of CRS ranging from anatomic abnormalities to polyposis. Unilateral polyps are less common than bilateral polyps and when seen should raise suspicion for other conditions such as carcinoma, inverting papilloma or allergic fungal sinusitis. In fungal infection or neoplasm, osseous destruction may be seen on sinus CT. MRI is indicated when fungal infection or neoplasm is suspected.

In CRS, nasal endoscopy and anterior rhinoscopy both offer direct visualization of sinusoidal mucosa. While anterior rhinoscopy allows for visualization of anterior ⅓ of nasal cavity, nasal endoscopy allows visualization of posterior nasal, nasopharynx, and often the sinus drainage pathways in the middle meatus and superior meatus. Nasal endoscopy also allows aspiration of nasal secretions for analysis and culture. In cases where suspicion for CRS is high, nasal endoscopy can be used alone without sinus CT for diagnosis. CT in these cases being reserved for complicated or prolonged clinical course (**Table 5**).

Modality	Method	Risk	Cost	Sensitivity
Nasal endoscopy	Direct visualization	Minimal	Moderate	Good
Anterior rhinoscopy	Direct visualization	Minimal	Minimal	Fair
CT scan	Radiographic	Radiation exposure	High	Excellent

Table 5.
Showing modality of diagnostics with associated cost, risk, and sensitivity.

9. Long term monitoring and prevention

Management of AVRS is supportive and focuses on symptom relief with analgesics or antipyretic drugs (NSAIDS, acetaminophen), decongestants (oxymetazoline), intranasal steroids (mometasone) and saline irrigation. AVRS is self-limited and typically peaks within 3 days then resolves within 10 to 14 days [5].

Management of ABRS also includes symptom relief with the same pharmacological therapy as AVRS. In addition to supportive treatment, antibiotic therapy also plays a role in treating ABRS. Antibiotics can either be started at time of diagnosis or after the watchful waiting period. If ABRS fail to improve after 7 days of the watchful waiting period, antibiotics should be started.

When antibiotics are used, first-line therapy is amoxicillin for 5–10 days. High dose amoxicillin is used to cover penicillin non susceptible *Streptococcus pneumoniae*. High dose amoxicillin with clavulanate is also used if bacterial resistance is suspected (antibiotic use in the past month, treatment failure or worsening of symptoms, high prevalence of resistance bacteria in the community), presence of moderate to severe infection (symptoms for extended time), presence of comorbidity (diabetes mellitus, immunocompromised, older than 65). Doxycycline or a respiratory fluoroquinolone (levofloxacin or moxifloxacin) is used in type I hypersensitivity penicillin-allergic patients [6].

When managing CRS and recurrent ARS, it is important to identify the risk factors that contribute to the persistence or recurrence of the illness since the burden of the comorbidities often decreases with prompt initiation of CRS therapy. Such risk factors/ comorbidities as already mentioned earlier in the chapter are asthma, cystic fibrosis, immunocompromised state, ciliary dyskinesia, or anatomic deformities. For instance, immunodeficiencies in IgA and IgG have been documented in patients with CRS and recurrent ARS. In such cases quantitative immunoglobulin measurements may be considered in patients presenting with CRS and recurrent ARS, especially in those that have failed aggressive management or when sinusitis is associated with bronchiectasis or otitis media. Chronic antibiotic therapy or intranasal steroids have not shown benefits in reducing episodes of recurrent ARS. Patients presenting with recurrent ARS should undergo allergy testing and/or immunologic testing to test for coexisting allergic rhinitis or immunodeficiency. Management of recurrent ARS in the setting of these comorbidities should focus on treating the coexisting illness. Sinus surgery is also an option in such patients.

Treatment of CRS, like AVRS and ABRS, relies on symptom control with saline irrigation. Topical intranasal steroids such as mometasone also play a role in treating CRS due to their anti-inflammatory properties and for symptom relief. These benefits have been seen especially in CRS with polyps. Topical nasal steroids should be used for at least 8–12 weeks to show benefits. If no response is seen within 3 months, a short course of oral corticosteroids can be initiated. As for antibiotics, macrolides where found to be beneficial in CRS with polyps due to their anti-inflammatory properties.

10. Future research

Differentiating AVRS from ABRS clinically can be difficult. Positive sinus aspiration and culture would be helpful in diagnosis ABRS but also problematic due to contaminants from the nose.

Efficacy of antibiotic therapy for ABRS could be further analyzed via pre and post therapy sinus cultures which may open the door for the use of endoscopic middle meatus cultures or sinus puncture. These invasive methods are indicated for patients who failed to respond to first line and second line therapy. It is recommended to perform sinus aspiration (rather than nasopharyngeal swab) since it was shown to be the most accurate. Endoscopically directed cultures of the middle meatus are also acceptable although less accurate than sinus cultures obtained by sinus puncture.

High dose amoxicillin-clavulanate is used to treat penicillin non-susceptible *Streptococcus pneumoniae*, severe infection etc. But more studies are warranted to compare the efficacy of respiratory fluoroquinolones over that of high dose amoxicillin-clavulanate.

Macrolides, second and third generation oral cephalosporins and TMP/SMX are not recommended as antibiotics therapy due to high rates of resistance among *Streptococcus pneumoniae*. If an oral cephalosporin must be used, third generation in combination with clindamycin is recommended. Among the third-generation oral cephalosporin, cefditoren seems to be the one with the best activity against penicillin non susceptible *Streptococcus pneumoniae*. Doxycycline on the other hand can be used as an alternative to amoxicillin-clavulanate for adults at low risk of penicillin non susceptible *Streptococcus pneumoniae*. More randomized controlled trials are warranted to assess efficacy of doxycycline and cefditoren.

Resistance patterns vary based on geography, but also based on the time of the surveillance study. It is necessary that antimicrobial susceptibility profiles of pathogens in questions be studied nationally, locally, and temporally.

The recommended duration of antibiotic treatment in adults is 5–10 days, which is somewhat arbitrary. Most clinical trials have excluded severely ill patients and included patients with maxillary sinusitis without involvement of other sinuses. More research is needed for the optimal duration of treatment.

Conflict of interest

Authors declares no conflict of interest.

Abbreviations

ARS	Acute rhinosinusitis
AVRS	Acute viral rhinosinusitis
ABRS	Acute bacterial rhinosinusitis
CRS	Chronic rhinosinusitis
CT	Computed tomography
NSAIDs	Non-steroidal ant-inflammatory
URTI	Upper respiratory tract infection

Author details

Jana I. Preis[1*†], Anna W. Maro[2†], Sophie Hurez[2†] and Sneha Pusapati[2†]

1 Division of Infectious Diseases and Clinical Epidemiology, Brooklyn VA Medical Center, SUNY Downstate Health Science University, Brooklyn, New York, USA

2 SUNY Downstate Health Science University, Brooklyn, New York, USA

*Address all correspondence to: info@idcq.org

† These authors contributed equally.

References

[1] Scheid D. & Hamm R : Acute Bacterial Rhinosinusitis in Adults. *American Family Physician,* 2004 1 ;70 (9) : 1685-1692, https://www.aafp.org/afp/2004/1101/p1685.html

[2] Mr Gray's Illustrations, Radiopaedia.org, Gray's Anatomy 20th US edition. https://radiopaedia.org/cases/nose-and-nasal-cavities?lang=us

[3] https://www.uptodate.com/contents/acute-sinusitis-and-rhinosinusitis-in-adults-clinical-manifestations-anddiagnosis?search=epidemiology%20of%20rhinosinusitis&source=search_result&selectedTitle=1~150&usage_type=default&display_rank=1

[4] Jaume F, Valls-Mateus M & Mullol J : Common Cold and Acute Rhinosinusitis, 2020 ; *Current allergy and Asthma Reports,* Article number :28 (2020) https://link.springer.com/article/10.1007/s11882-020-00917-5#Sec3. DOI: 10.1007/s11882-020-00917-5 PMID: 32495003 PMCID: PMC7266914

[5] Aring A, Chan M : Acute Rhinosinusitis in Adults ; *American Family Physician* https://www.aafp.org/afp/2011/0501/p1057.html

[6] Chow A, Benninger S, Brook I : IDSA Clinical Practice Guideline for Acute Bacterial Rhinosinusitis in Children and Adults. *Clinical Infectious Disease*, 2012, Vol 54, pages e72-e112, https://doi.org/10.1093/cid/cis370

Chapter 3

Posterior Ethmoidal Artery: Surgical Anatomy and Variations

Smail Kharoubi

Abstract

The posterior ethmoidal artery is a collateral of the ophthalmic artery and participates in the vascularization of the nasal cavities. It is an important landmark in endonasal surgery with complex orbital contents relationships. We recognize many anatomical and functional varieties. This chapter proposes to present a classic descriptive anatomical study but also a modern radiological and endoscopic study of the posterior ethmoidal artery. It also proposes to present a description of some pathologies associated with this artery, particulary posterior epistaxis and other vascular disorders. The surgical procedur to access to posterior ethmoidal artery, external or endoscopic approach of the posterior ethmoidal artery will be described.

Keywords: posterior ethmoidal artery, epistaxis, ligation posterior ethmoidal artery, skull base surgery, complication endonasal surgery

1. Introduction

Posterior ethmoidal artery is a branch of the ophthalmic artery and participates in the vascularization of the upper part of the nasal cavities, dura mater, ethmoid and sphenoidal sinuses. it often leads into a bony canal and is 14 mm from the anterior ethmoidal artery and 7 mm from the optic foramen.

The posterior ethmoidal artery is involved in several nasosinusal and base of skull pathology or abnormalities. It may be responsible for persistant epistaxis requiring specific treatment or producing aneurysm lesion with its compressive and hemorrhagic complications.

Imaging (CT-scan of the facial mass, arteriography) facilitate its study as well as its bone canal and its orbital spheno ethmoidal reports.

Ligation of the posterior ethmoidal artery allows effective hemostasis during intractable epistaxis or as a preventive procedure in surgery of skull base meningiomas.

2. Embryology

The arterial blood supply to the orbit depends on that of the cerebral arteries. Since the work of Padget [1], we admit that the six aortic arches, connecting the ventral and dorsal ipsilateral aortas, appear very early.

The internal carotid arises from the 3rd arch and gives rise to the two primary ophthalmic arteries, ventral and dorsal.

Ophtalmic artery will give anterior ethmoidal artery, posterior ethmoidal artery and sometimes middle ethmoidal artery.

3. Anatomy

3.1 Origin

The posterior ethmoidal artery is a small collateral branch of the ophthalmic artery that leaves the orbit (posterior third of the orbit) through the posterior orbital canal and is found at the junction of the roof of the sphenoid and posterior ethmoid sinuses (**Figures 1** and **2**).

Anatomical variations at the origin occur more frequently in the posterior ethmoidal artery (86%). Many anatomical variations frequently occur at the origin of the PEA The posterior ethmoidal artery can also originate from the third part of the ophthalmic artery (5%), or from the second part of the ophthalmic artery (5%). It may have its origin in the AEA and also in the middle meningeal.

3.2 Course

From the posterior orbital canal the artery goes up and back.

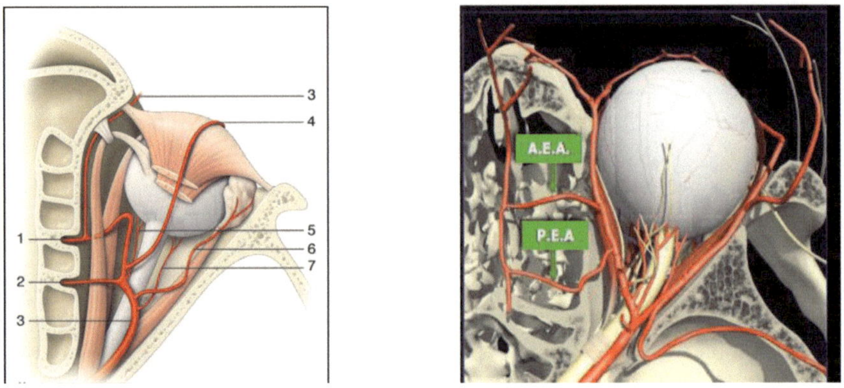

Figure 1.
Intra orbital ophtalmic artery: 1. anterior ethmoidal artery (AEA); 2. posterior ethmoidal artery (PEA) 3. ophtalmic artery; 4. supra orbital artery; 5. medialy long ciliary artery; 6.lacrymal artery; 7. lateral long ciliary artery. (Iconography - Ducasse. A Ref. [2]).

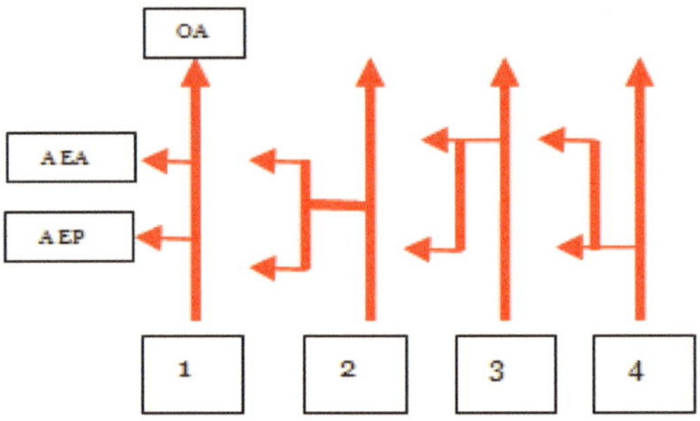

Figure 2.
Anatomic variability of origin of ethmoidal arteries. OA: ophtalmic artery AEA: anterior ethmoidal artery AEP: posterior ethmoidal artery. 1: independent origin of ethmoidal arteries. 2: common origin (single trunk) of anterior and posterior artery. 3: posterior ethmoidal artery origin from anterior ethmoidal artery. 4: anterior ethmoidal artery origin from posterior ethmoidal artery.

It runs between the rectus superior and the superior oblique muscle and then emerges from the myofascial cone of the orbit to finally pass perpendicular to the medial wall and enter the posterior ethmoidal canal.

Posterior ethmoidal artery into its canal presents a more horizontal orientation than that of the anterior ethmoidal artery with an entry angle into the skull base of between 0° and 18°.

The posterior ethmoidal artery is smaller than the anterior ethmoidal artery, usually less than 1 mm, which makes its identification difficult in CT studies. Its size is usually inversely proportional to that of the anterior ethmoidal artery.

The intra orbital part has a 0.66 ± 0.21 mm diameter and 0.63 ± 0.19 on the left.

The intracranial part has a 0.45 ± 0.12 mm (range, 0.32 to 0.57 mm) diameter. Tomkinson et al. they could identify the PEA in only 14/40 nasal fossae [3].

Posterior ethmoidal artery runs very close to the optic nerve: the distance between the two structures is variable and can range from 4 to 16 mm (**Table 1**) (**Figure 3**).

3.3 Termination

It ends in the posterior part of the lateral wall of the nasal cavity.

In medial wall of nasal cavity (septum) posterior ethmoidal artery contribuate to kisselbach area with superior labial, anterior ethmoidal and naso palatine artery (**Figure 4**).

3.4 Branche

- anterior tract olfactif artery.
- accessory posterior olfactory artery (**Figure 5**).

Author	Distance	Measurement
Cankal et al., 2004 [4]	From nasion to PEF	46.3 mm (range 38–55 mm)
	From optic foramen to PEF	6.7 mm (range 4–16 mm)
Caliot et al., 1995 [5]	From AEF to PEF	10–15 mm
	From optic foramen to PEF	5 mm

PEA: posterior ethmoidal artery. PEF: posterior ethmoidal foramen. AEF: anterior ethmoidal foramen.

Table 1.
Anatomical landmarks in the literature for identifying the PEA.

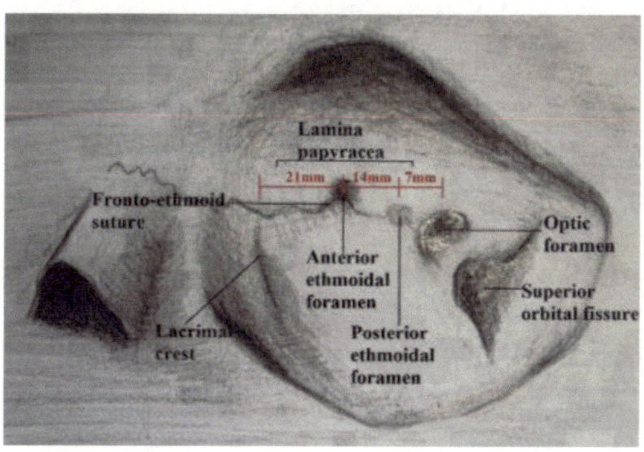

Figure 3.
The medial wall of the orbit. The fronto ethmoidal suture guides the sub periorbital dissection to the anterior and posterior ethmoidal foramen. The main bony landmarks are highlighted. (Iconography - Cecchini. G Ref. [6]).

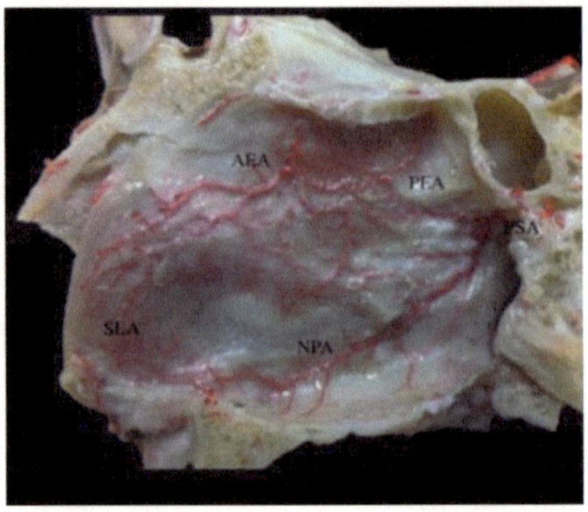

Figure 4.
Nasal septum vascularisation. NPA nasopalatine artery, SLA superior labial artery, AEA anterior ethmoidal artery, PEA posterior ethmoidal artery, PSA posterior septal artery. (Iconography-Gras-Cabrerizo. JR Ref. [7]).

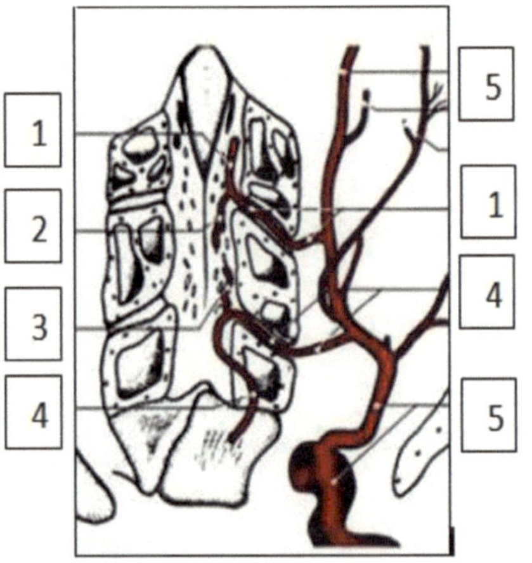

Figure 5.
Branch of posterior ethmoidal artery. 1: anterior ethmoidal artery. 2: anterior tract olfactif artery. 3: accessory olfactif artery. 4: posterior ethmoidal artery. 5: orbitary artery. (Iconography - Ducasse. A Ref. [2]).

3.5 Anastomoses

We can found some anastomoses of posterior ethmoidal artery with septal artery, lateral nasal artery and anterior ethmoidal artery (**Table 2**).

3.6 Supply

It irrigates the sphenoid sinus and the dura mater which covers the riddled blade of the ethmoid.

The posterior ethmoidal arteries ran anteriorly and inferiorly divided through the crista galli suture to supply the anterior ethmoidal territory.

There is often a meningeal branch to the dura mater while it is still contained within the cranium. This artery supplies:

- the posterior ethmoidal.
- dura mater of the anterior canal fossa.

INTERNAL CAROTID ARTERY	**EXTERNAL CAROTID ARTERY**
↓	↓
OPHTALMIC ARTERY	**MAXILLARY ARTERY**
↓	↓
CENTRAL RETINAL ARTERY	**SPHENOPALATINE ARTERY**
POSTERIOR CILIARY ARTERIES	↓
LACRIMAL ARTERY	
MUSCULAR ARTERIES	
SUPRAORBITAL ARTERY	
POSTERIOR ETHMOIDAL ARTERY ↔	LATERAL NASAL ARTERY
ANTERIOR ETHMOIDAL ARTERY ↔	SEPTAL ARTERY
PALPEBRAL ARTERIES	
DORSAL NASAL ARTERY	
SUPRATROCHLEAR ARTERY	

Table 2.
Diagramm anastomoses posterior ethmoidal artery.

- the upper part of the nasal mucosa of the nasal septum and it anastomoses with the sphenopalatine artery.

4. Endoscopic anatomy

The identification of the posterior ethmoidal artery during endonasal surgery is an important step and allows an adapted hemostasis. The first step being a regulated ethmoidectomy which begins with the identification of the anterior ethmoidal artery (sometimes in a bony canal) then the posterior ethmoidal artery further back.

The posterior ethmoidal artery is the landmark access to the sphenoidal sinus (**Figures 6–8**).

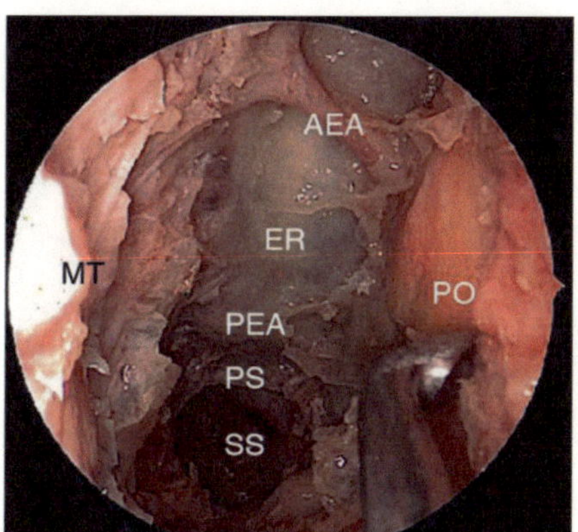

Figure 6.
*Endoscopic view of the left anterior skull base. (*AEA *anterior ethmoidal artery,* ER *ethmoid roof,* PEA *posterior ethmoidal artery,* PS, *planum sphenoidale,* SS *sphenoid sinus,* PO *periorbita,* MT *middle turbinate). (Iconography - McClurg. SW Ref. [8]).*

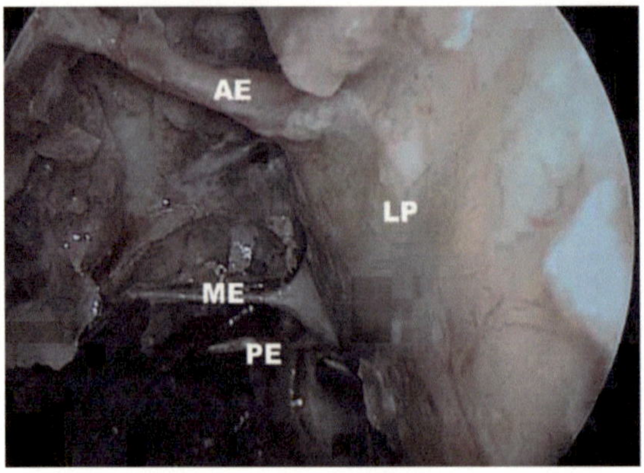

Figure 7.
*Endoscopic view of the left nasal cavity. (*AE *anterior ethmoidal artery,* ME *middle ethmoidal artery,* PE *posterior ethmoidal artery,* LP *lamina papyracea bone* PS, *planum sphenoidale,* SS *sphenoid sinus,* PO *periorbita,* MT *middle turbinate). (Iconography - Kürşat Gökcan. M Ref. [9]).*

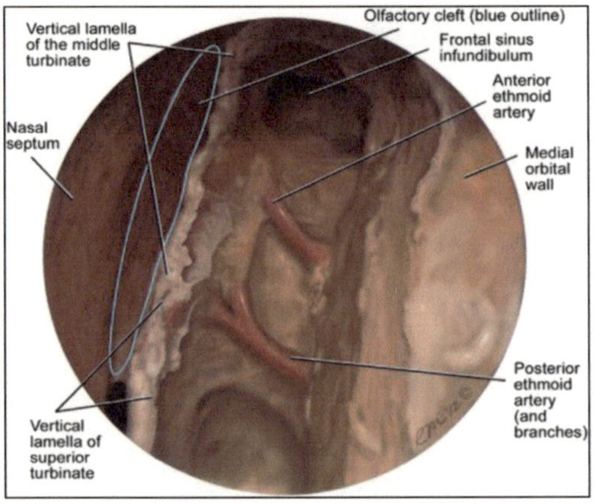

Figure 8.
The bony canal of anterior and posterior ethmoidal artery is seen through the ethmoid roof traveling from the orbit to the cribriform plate. (Iconography - Casiano Roy. R Ref. [10]).

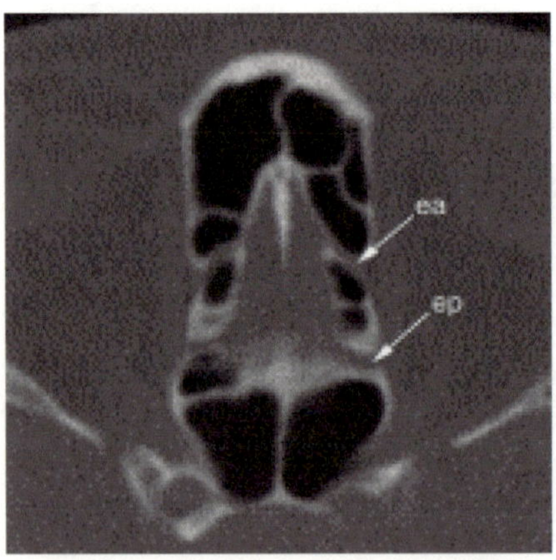

Figure 9.
Computed tomography axial view anterior and posterior ethmoidal arteries in canals ea: anterior ethmoidal artery, ep: posterior ethmoidal artery.

5. Radiology

The ethmoidal arteries more easily identifiable on the axial view. CT-scan (with contrast) is a best exam from identifing ethmoidal arteries (anterior, middle and posterior arteries).

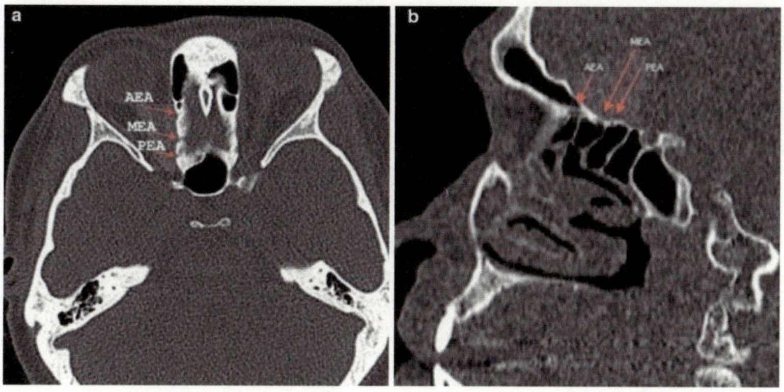

Figure 10.
CT scan axial (a) and saggital (b) view: ethmoidal arteries (anterior, medial and posterior ethmoidal arteries). (Iconography - Kho. JPY Ref. [11]).

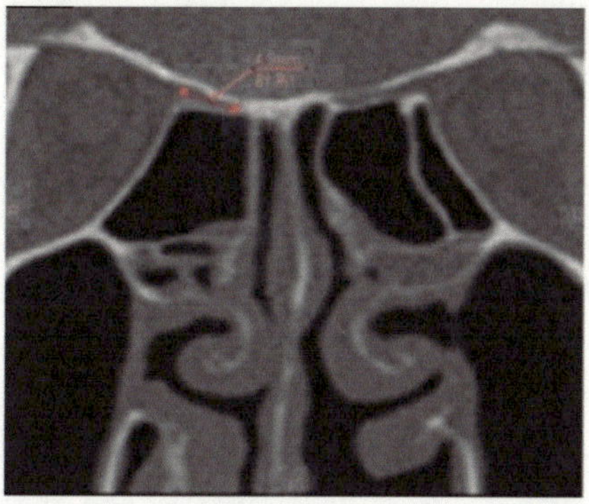

Figure 11.
Length of the PEA (4,9mm) exposed in the ethmoid cells on coronal CT scan. (Iconography - Yamamoto. H Ref. [12]).

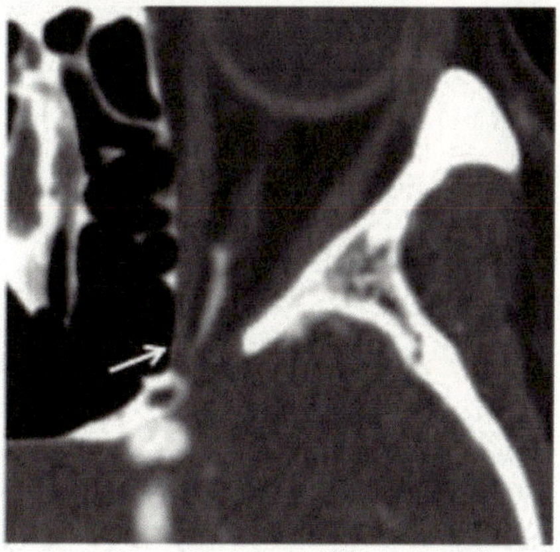

Figure 12.
Axial view of computed tomography scan with contrast enhancement revealed the PEA passing through the medial wall of the orbit and into the posterior ethmoidal sinus. (Iconography - Casiano Roy. R Ref. [10]).

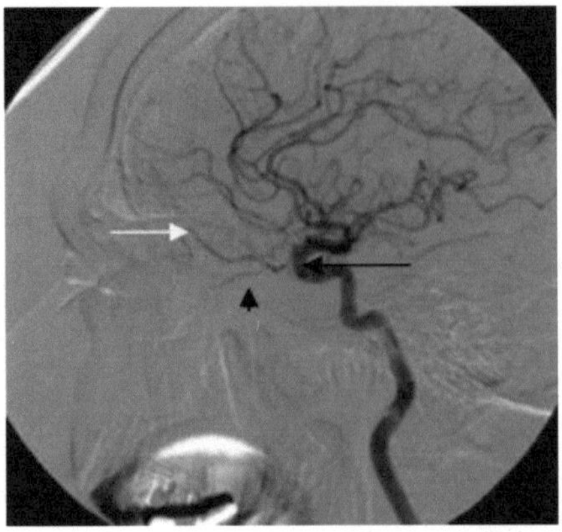

Figure 13.
Arteriography: Ethmoide vascularization by branches from the left ophtalmic artery. Black arrow: ophtalmic artery. White arrow: anterior ethmoidal artery. Black head arrow: posterior ethmoidal artery. (Iconography - Giuseppe Greco. M Ref. [13]).

The posterior ethmoidal artery usually crosses within the ethmoidal roof, in front of the most superior aspect of the anterior wall of the sphenoid sinus. In 25–50%, the corticated sulcus of this artery is identifiable on the coronal CT examination (**Figures 9–13**).

6. Pathology

6.1 Aneurysm of the posterior ethmoidal artery

6.1.1 Moyamoya

The Moyamoya disease is a cerebrovascular condition that predisposes patients to stroke in association with progressive stenosis of the intracranial internal carotid arteries and their proximal branches. Furthermore in moyamoya patients, intracranial aneurysms are known to occur at the level of the polygon of Willis (often in the vertebra-basilar circulation), more rarely on the basal ganglia arteries or on anterior or posterior choroidal arteries.

One exceptionally case of posterior ethmoidal artery anevrysm by moyamoya was repported (**Figure 14**) [14].

6.1.2 Post traumatic aneuvrysm

Head trauma or skull base fracture can to induce anevrysmal lesion with some arteries like posterior ethmoidal artery.

6.2 Arteriovenous malformation and posterior ethmoidal artery

In some cases arteriovenous malformationcan to be feding by a posterior ethmoidal artery. Computer tomograhy and arteriography facilitited the diagnosis and recognize their support artery [15].

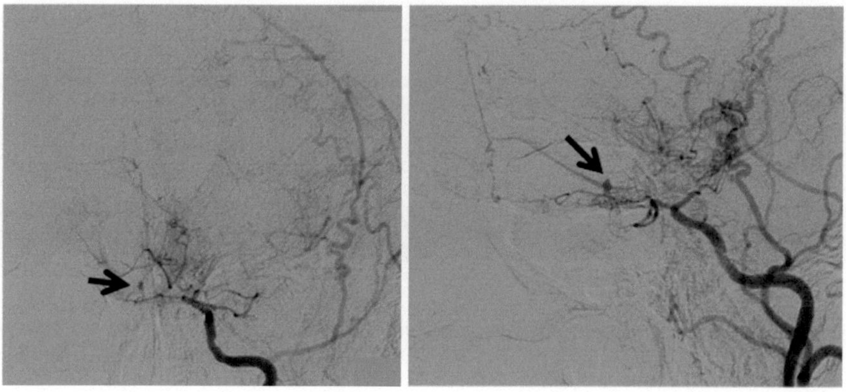

Figure 14.
Front view and Oblique view. Aneurysm of the right posterior ethmoidal artery fed by the left ophthalmic artery (black arrow). (Iconography - Mélota. A Ref. [14]).

6.3 Epistaxis

Clinical specificity: posterior and superior issue bleeding in nasal cavity.

- When bleeding seems to come from the roof of the nasal cavity, it is important to identify the ethmoid arteries always bearing in mind the possible existence of anomalous courses.

- Posterior bleeding (10% of epistaxis) usually originates from the spheno palatine artery or from its branches or, more rarely, from the anterior or posterior ethmoid arteries, branches of the ophthalmic artery [8, 16].

Failure of ligation of the sphenopalatine artery in profuse and recurrent posterior epistaxis will be indicate ligation of the anterior and posterior ethmoidal arteries.

7. Surgery of posterior ethmoidal artery

Elective ligation of anterior and posterior ethmoidal arteries is indicates for extended endonasal procedures when control of these vascular structures is an essential component of the procedure, such as in endoscopic craniofacial resections.

Rarely, intractable or traumatic epistaxis requires ligation of these arteries, but this is probably best managed externally with endoscopic assistance.

7.1 Extra cranial open bilateral anterior ANS posterior ethmoidal artery ligation

- Lynch incision.

- exposure down to the perioteum of the medial orbital walls.

- the frontoethmoidal suture is followed bluntly for about 22 mm posterior to the lacrimal crest and the posterior ethmoidal artery is encountered about 15 mm posterior to the anterior ethmoidal artery.

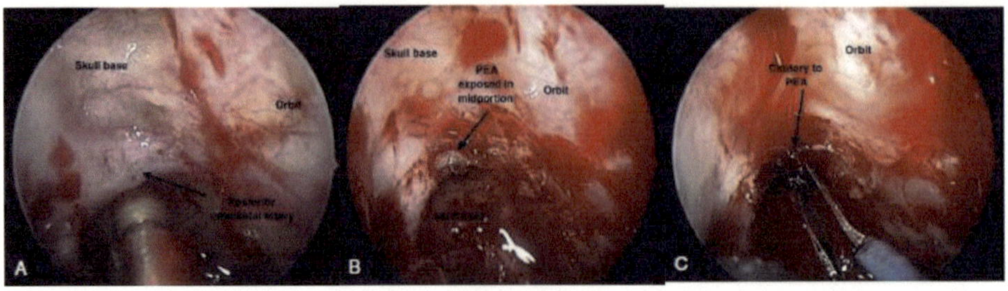

Figure 15.
Posterior ethmoidal artery: endoscopic approach. A: posterior ethmoidal artery in osseus canal. B: posterior ethmoidal artery (PEA) exposed in midportion. C: cauterisation of posterior ethmoidal artery. (Iconography - Naidoo. Y Ref. [17]).

7.2 Extra cranial transcaruncular approach

- incision lateral to the caroncule.
- identifying the lacrimal fossa.
- following the avascular facial plans posteromedially to the frontoethmoidal suture.
- the periosteum is incised bilaterally to allow a posterior sub periosteal dissection trajectory to the anterior ethmoidal arteries.

7.3 Endoscopic transnasal approach

The endoscopic approach of the ethmoidal arteries requires a good learning of endoscopic ethmoidectomy. The identification of the ethmoidal roof does not present any specificity like with conventional ethmoidectomy.

If you will to recognize the posterior ethmoidal artery, you must expose the posterior spheno ethmoidal region. The 0° optic is generally used: the region of the posterior ethmoidal artery being almost in the axis of the nasal cavity, it is quite easy to use a bipolar endonasal coagulant forceps (Dessi tool) for coagulation if the artery is easy viewable (whithout to embedding in the ethmoidal roof). identification of anterior ethmoidal artery is possible by following the ethmoidal roof to the fronto ethmoidal recess. In the majority of cases (83%), the artery is visible by this way (**Figure 15**) [18].

7.4 Endovascular approach

Because of the abundant anastomoses among anterior ethmoidal artery, posterior ethmoidal artery, collateral branches from Middle meningeal artery and Internal carotid artery, endovascular embolization puts the ophthalmic artery and vision at risk, so it is not recommandable to doing or choise embolisation of ethmoidal arteries.

8. Conclusion

The posterior ethmoidal artery branch of the ophthalmic artery is an anatomical, endoscopic and radiological entity very important to know in diagnosis, pathology and surgery of nasal and para nasal diseases.

The complete analysis of this anatomical structure will help and facilitate medical and surgical practice.

Conflict of interest

No conflict of interest.

Author details

Smail Kharoubi
Department of ENT, Chu Annaba, Faculty of Medicine, University of Badji Mokhtar, Annaba, Algeria

*Address all correspondence to: smail.kharoubi17@gmail.com

References

[1] Padget.DH. The development of the cranial arteries in the human embryo. Carnegie institution of Washington. Contrib Embryol 1948;32:205–61.

[2] Ducasse.A, Larré.I Anatomy and vascularization of the orbit. EMC Elsevier Paris 2020 21-006-A-10 19 pages.

[3] Tomkinson.A, Roblin.DG, Flanagan. P et al. "Patterns of hospital attendance with epistaxis". Rhinology 1997 vol. 35, pp. 129–135.

[4] Cankal F, Apaydin N, Acar HI, Elhan A, Tekdemir I, Yurdakul M, et al Evaluation of the anterior and posterior ethmoidal canal by computed tomography. Clin Radiol 2004 59:1034–1040. doi: 10.1016/j.crad.2004.04.016.

[5] Caliot.P, Plessis. JL, Midy.D, Poirier. M, Ha.JC The intraorbital arrangement of the anterior and posterior ethmoidal foramina. Surg Radiol Anat 1995 17:29–33. doi: 10.1007/BF01629496.

[6] Cecchini.G Anterior and Posterior Ethmoidal Artery Ligation in Anterior Skull Base Meningiomas:A Review on Microsurgical Approaches. World Neurosurg 2015 84 1[4] october : 1161-1165. doi: 10.1016/j. wneu.2015.06.005. Epub 2015 Jun 11.

[7] Gras-Cabrerizo.JR, Garcı'a-Garrigo's. E, Montserrat-Gili.JR, Juan R. Gras-Albert.JR, Mirapeix-Lucas.R And Al. Anatomical Correlation Between Nasal Vascularisationand the Design of the Endonasal Pedicle Flaps. Indian J Otolaryngol Head Neck Surg (Jan–Mar 2018) 70(1):167–173. doi.org/10.1007/s12070-017-1197-z.

[8] McClurg.WMS, Carrau.R Endoscopic management of posterior epistaxis:a review. Acta otorhinolaryngol ital 2014; 34:1-8.

[9] Kürşat Gökcan.M,Beton.S,Küçük.B. Endoscopic Skull Base Surgery: Anatomical Basis of Skull Base Approaches. Springer Nature Switzerland AG 2020 663 C. Cingi, N. Bayar Muluk (eds.), *All Around the Nose*. doi.org/10.1007/978-3-030-21217-9_75.

[10] Casiano Roy.R, Herzallah Islam.R, Anstead Amy.S, et al Advanced endoscopic sinonasal dissection, in Endoscopic Sinonasal Dissection Guide, New York: Thieme 2011.

[11] Kho.JPY, Tang.IP,Tan.KS, Koa.AJ, Prepageran.N Radiological Study of the Ethmoidal Arteries in the Nasal Cavity and Its Pertinence to the Endoscopic Surgeon. Indian J Otolaryngol Head Neck Surg (November 2019) 71 (Suppl 3):S1994–S1999. doi.org/10.1007/s12070-018-1415-3 Rajagopalan1

[12] Yamamoto.H, Nomura.K ,Hidaka.H, Katori.Y,Yoshida.N Anatomy of the posterior and middle ethmoidal arteries via computed tomography SAGE Open Med 2018 Volume 6 1–7. doi: 10.1177/2050312118772473.eCollection 2018.

[13] Giuseppe Greco.M, Mattioli.F, Alberici.MP,Presutti.L Recurrent Massive Epistaxis from an Anomalous Posterior Ethmoid Artery Case Rep Otolaryngol Volume 2016, 1-4. doi.org/10.1155/2016/8504348.

[14] Mélota.A, Chazota.JV, Troudea.L, De la Rosaa.S, Brunelb.H,Rochea.PH Ruptured posterior ethmoidal artery aneurysm and Moyamoya disease in an adult patient. Case report. Neurochirurgie 2016 62 171–173. doi: 10.1016/j.neuchi.2016.04.001. Epub 2016 May 25.

[15] Fritz .Wz , Klein.HJ, Schmidt.K. Arteriovenous malformation of the posterior ethmoidal artery as an unusual cause of amaurosis fugax. The

ophthalmic steal syndrome. J Clin Neuroophthalmol . 1989 Sep;9(3):165-8. doi: 10.3109/01658108909010470.

[16] Hayashi Y, Kita D, Iwato M, Nakanishi S, Hamada. Massive He morrhage from the Posterior Ethmoidal Artery during Transsphenoidal Surgery: Report of 2 Cases. J.Turk Neurosurg. 2015;25(5):804-7. doi: 10.5137/1019-5149.JTN.11013-14.0.

[17] Naidoo.Y, Wormald.PJ Endoscopic and Open Anterior/Posterior Ethmoid Artery Ligation. Chapter 5 . In Atlas of Endoscopic Sinus and Skull Base Surgery 2nd Edition- Nithin Adappa James Palmer Alexander Chiu. Elsevier Editor.2018.

[18] Erdogmus.S , Govsa.F "The anatomic landmarks of ethmoidal arteries for the surgical approaches," J Craniofac Surg, 2006 vol. 17, no. 2, pp. 280–285. doi: 10.1097/00001665-200603000-00014.

Chapter 4

Paranasal Sinuses Anatomy and Anatomical Variations

Hardip Singh Gendeh and Balwant Singh Gendeh

Abstract

Anatomical variations of the sinuses are common and may lead to obstruction to the ventilation and drainage of the sinuses. This may lead to osteomeatal complex disease refractory to medications. A preoperative CT of the paranasal sinuses acts as road map guide to identify vital anatomical variations and its relationship to the orbit, skull base, neurological and vascular structures, to prevent iatrogenic injuries. To control intraoperative bleeding, it is critical to identify the anterior and posterior ethmoidal artery indentations and sphenopalatine artery in the anterior and lateral nasal walls. It is essential for the surgeon to familiarize with the anatomy of the ethmoid region, lateral nasal wall, sphenoid sinus, sella and parasellar region and pterygopalatine/infratemporal fossa before embarking on these approaches. The advent of CT scans and state-of-the-art FESS instrumentation has made surgery of the paranasal sinuses less of a mystery for the surgeon. Therefore, identifying and addressing these anatomical variations during FESS is crucial in restoring ventilation and drainage.

Keywords: paranasal sinus, anatomy, anatomical variations, endoscopic surgery

1. Introduction

The birth of Endoscopic Sinus Surgery (ESS) in the early 1900 in Graz, Austria, under the teachings of Messerklinger has led to an understanding of the drainage of the paranasal sinuses. Messerklinger introduced the world to tailored endoscopic sinus surgery owing to his work in the frontal recess and ethmoidal infundibulum for drainage of sinuses [1, 2]. This was then popularized by Stammberger and Kennedy with the term functional endoscopic sinus surgery (FESS) being introduced. FESS involves ventilating and draining of the sinuses with preservation of the mucosa [3]. In the advent of FESS, nasal radiograph was constrained in identifying anatomical variations of the sinuses and paranasal sinuses. The use of high-resolution computed tomography (CT) scans with 2–3 millimeters slices has allowed for better spatial resolution of the anatomical structures.

Prior to performing an ESS, one must obtain a high-resolution CT of the sinuses and paranasal sinuses for diagnosis and to identify anatomical variations present, both of which are essential for surgical planning. This is useful to direct the course of the endoscopic operation in relieving obstructions and drainage of the sinuses. The surgeon will also become aware of anatomical variations such as a low-lying base of skull to prevent iatrogenic injuries, reduce complications, and avoid failure of surgery. Coronal images are particularly important and give information of the vast anatomy of the paranasal sinuses.

Prior to leaping into the radiological images of such variations, one must first understand the development of the sinuses to appreciate the acceptable differences between a pediatric and adult sinus. Both the maxillary and ethmoidal sinuses are present at birth. The maxillary sinuses reach adult size by 15 years, while the ethmoidal sinuses are earlier at 12 years. The maxillary sinus can be appreciated radiologically at several months after birth and ethmoidal later at approximately 12 months [4]. The frontal and sphenoid sinuses are not present and begin development after birth. The frontal sinuses invaginate into the frontal recess from the age of 4 and continues to expand until the age of 20. The sphenoid sinus attains its full size by 15 years [4].

These anatomical variations may obstruct the drainage and ventilation of the sinuses resulting in sinusitis with or without headaches [5]. Anatomical variations of the middle meatus such as paradoxical middle turbinate, pneumatization and Haller's cells are the most common. This may lead to osteomeatal complex (OMC) diseases and will be required to be addressed if symptoms are persistent. O'Brien et al. 2016 have suggested a mnemonic CLOSE: cribriform plate, lamina papyracea, onodi cell, sphenoid sinus pneumatization, and ethmoidal artery (anterior) for critical structures that are often overlooked and underreported [6].

Variations in anatomy are more of a rule than an exception. Nature has customized different anatomies for every individual. Therefore, one must be aware of these possible variations before any surgical interventions. Air in the nose and paranasal sinuses acts as natural contrast; therefore, CT scan in bone and soft tissue windows is sufficient to diagnose anatomical variations and pathology in most cases of chronic rhinosinusitis. Although useful for a quick identification of pertinent variations, this chapter will introduce you to further variations that one may encounter when dealing with the sinuses and paranasal sinuses.

2. Nasal septum

The nasal septum forms the medial wall and separates the left and right nasal cavities, respectively. It also provides projection to the nose. It consists of three parts being the anterior cartilaginous septum formed by the quadrangular cartilage; posterior perpendicular plate of the ethmoid consisting of the perpendicular plate of ethmoid and vomer; and the most anterior membranous septum in between the quadrangular cartilage and the columella [7].

2.1 Nasal septal deviation

A deviated septum refers to a septal divergent from the midline (**Figure 1**). In general terms, an anterior deviation refers to the cartilaginous septum, while posterior involves the bony septum. Deviated nasal septum may cause compression and lateralization of the ipsilateral middle turbinate, often obstructing the ipsilateral OMC (**Figure 1**). This may lead to OMC disease causing obstruction to the drainage of the frontal, maxillary, and anterior ethmoidal sinus. Septal deviations may occur up to 36 and 4% of births having anterior cartilage deformity believed to be due to maxillary molding from pressure exerted within the birth canal [8, 9]. Shpilberg et al. 2014 reported 98.4% of 192 patients had a deviated nasal septum but 61.4% had a deviation more than minimal [10]. Hence, it is a common entity. The septum may be kinked to form a septal spur. Prominent septal spurs may have a dry mucosa and bleed due to increased surface area exposed to airflow. Some patients may have a mild deviation and are asymptomatic, while some may be symptomatic. Pathology

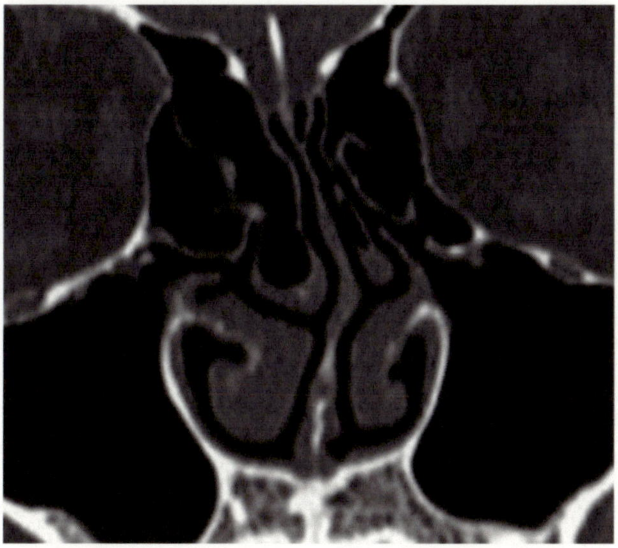

Figure 1.
A coronal view of CT of the paranasal sinus demonstrating a deviated left membranous nasal septum resulting in a hypoplastic left middle turbinate. The left middle turbinate is also pushed laterally and appears to be obstructing the left OMC. The contralateral right inferior turbinate is hypertrophied and larger than the left due to the larger right nasal cavity.

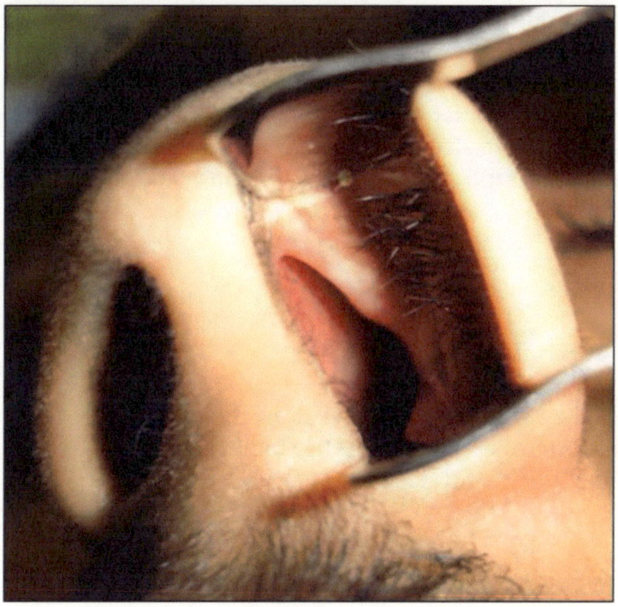

Figure 2.
Photograph showing an exposed anatomy of the normal nasal valve using thudicum's forcep. The nasal valve is boundary by the septum (medial), pyriform aperture (superior), upper lateral cartilage (lateral) and nasal floor (inferior).

in the nasal valve region (**Figure 2**) determines whether the patient will benefit from open (rhinoplasty) or closed septoplasty. Anterior nasal septal deviation involving the nasal valve causes valve collapse and airflow obstructions. These cohorts of patients will often benefit from a septorhinoplasty with a valve reconstruction [11].

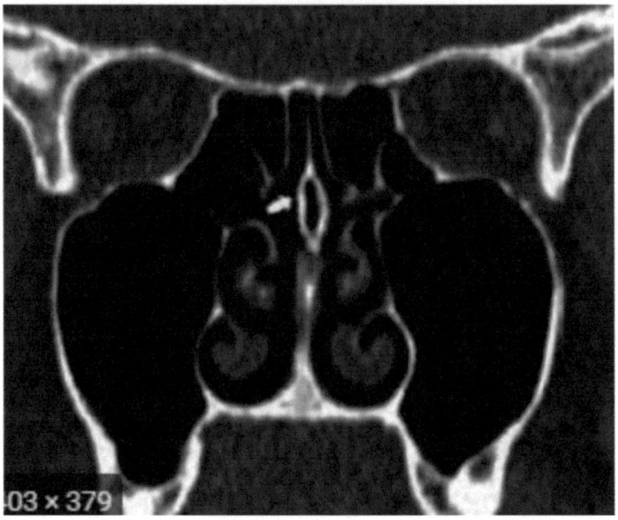

Figure 3.
A pneumatized cartilaginous nasal septum (white arrow) with surrounding calcification.

2.2 Pneumatized nasal septum

Pneumatization of the nasal septum is a rare entity (**Figure 3**). It may be due to trauma resulting in splitting of the cartilaginous or bony septum with a space in between. It may occur together with a nasal septal osteoma. It can be easily confused with a septal turbinate or septal polyp also known as intumescentia septi nasi anterior, which is a septal mucosal inflammation appreciated on endoscopic examination [12, 13]. Some have also referred to it as a pneumatized septal turbinate. It can be corrected with a septoplasty if there is significant obstruction.

3. Nasal turbinates

3.1 Hypoplasia of nasal turbinates

Hypoplasia of the turbinates is the result of the underdevelopment or reduced size due to reduced number of cells, in the small curved bones that extend horizontally along the lateral wall of the nose.

3.2 Pneumatization of the turbinates

Superior turbinate is a small bony projection in the lateral wall of the nose and forms the boundary of superior meatus and contributes to the formation of sphenoethmoidal recesses. Therefore, it plays a significant role in the drainage of the posterior ethmoidal and sphenoid sinuses. Pneumatization of the superior turbinate is rare and the incidence of it causing sinusitis is low compared with middle turbinate pneumatization (**Figure 4**). Extensive pneumatization of the middle turbinate (concha bullosa or bullous middle turbinate) is known to be one of the possible etiologic factors in nasal obstruction, recurrent sinusitis, and headaches (**Figure 5**). On the other hand, pneumatization of inferior turbinate is a very rarely encountered variation. Extensive turbinate pneumatization may cause turbinate enlargement and result in persistent nasal obstruction (**Figure 6**).

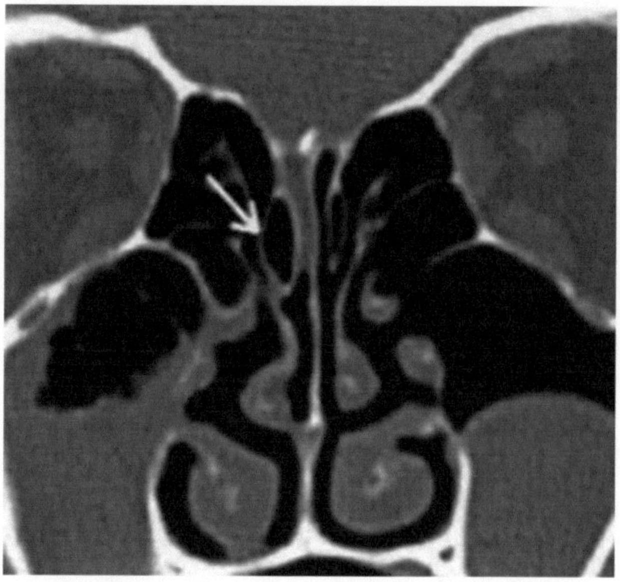

Figure 4.
A serial coronal CT scan of the paranasal sinuses showing pneumatization of right superior turbinate (arrow) with bilateral maxillary sinus pathology.

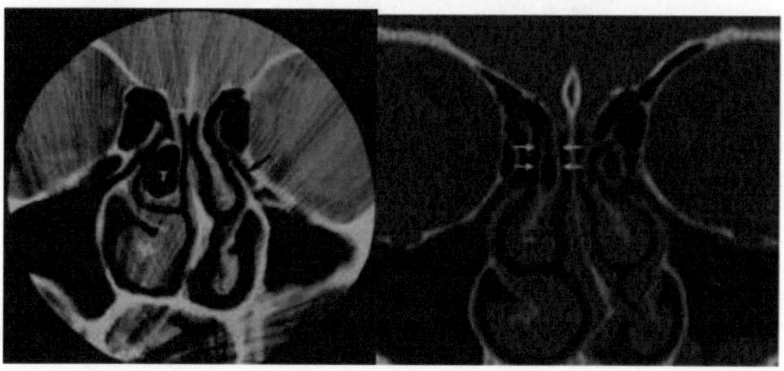

Figure 5.
Serial coronal CT scans of the paranasal sinuses showing a) pneumatization of right middle turbinate and B) pneumatized basal lamella (interlamellar cell of Grunwald) limited to vertical part of middle turbinate not causing narrowing of ostiomeatal complex.

3.3 Paradoxical turbinate

The superior, middle, and inferior turbinate (conchae) are present in the lateral wall of the nasal cavity. Paradoxical middle turbinate is a rare developmental condition and refers to an inferior medially curved middle turbinate edge with the concave surface facing the nasal septum and usually occurs bilaterally. Once again, it may impede sinus ventilation and drainage *via* the OMC, resulting in sinusitis (**Figure 7**).

3.4 Nasal septum turbinate

Nasal septal turbinate (NST) is structurally located in the anterior part of the septal part of nasal cavity and limits laterally the nasal valve (**Figure 8**). It presents a fusiform area of erectile tissue, similar in structure and function to nasal turbinate, and consists of mucosa, erectile tissue, blood vessels, and secretory glands. Its main

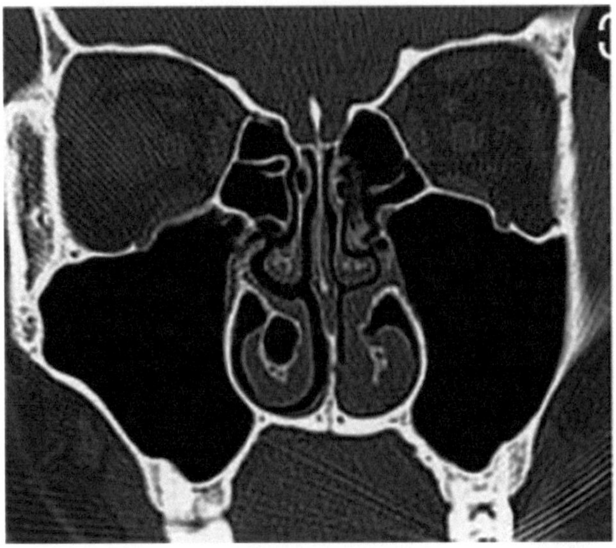

Figure 6.
A serial coronal CT scan of paranasal sinuses showing pneumatization of inferior turbinate.

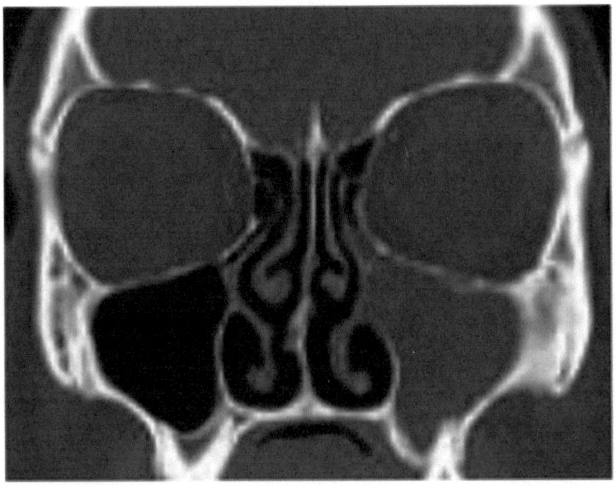

Figure 7.
A serial coronal CT scan of the paranasal sinuses showing paradoxical bilateral middle turbinates with an opaque left maxillary sinus.

function is to direct the airflow toward the nasal turbinate and the osteomeatal complex and humidification of air at the beginning of inspiration [14].

4. Uncinate process

4.1 Attachment of uncinate

The uncinate process (UP) is an important landmark for sinus surgery. It is a crescent-shaped bony projection forming a vital structure of the OMC unit, projecting from anterior superior in the posterior inferior direction. Its function is said to deflect and prevent contaminated inspired air from gaining access to the maxillary, anterior ethmoidal, and frontal sinus which it drains. The hiatus semilunaris, a two-dimensional structure, is bordered by the uncinate anterior

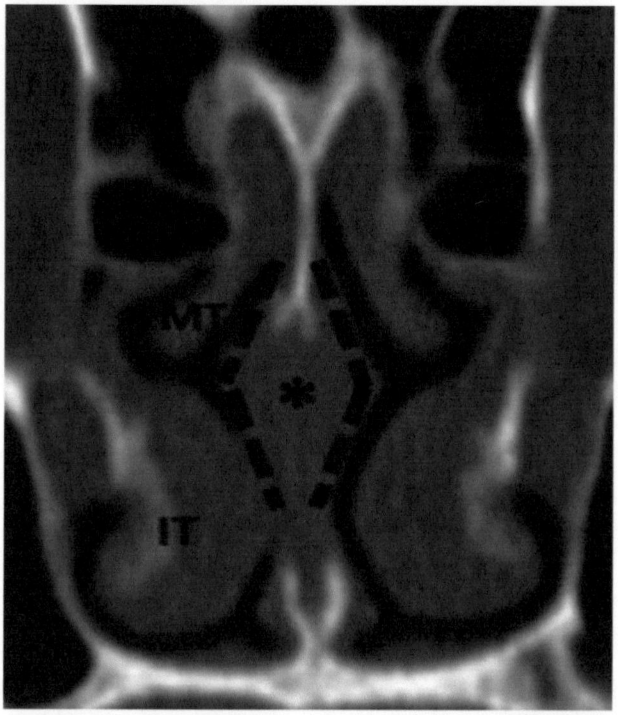

Figure 8.
A serial coronal CT scan of the paranasal sinuses showing nasal septum turbinate (asterisk).

inferiorly and ethmoidal bulla posterior superiorly. The hiatus semilunaris continues laterally to form the ethmoidal infundibulum, which is a three-dimensional conical structure with its apex lying laterally to form the maxillary sinus drainage pathway. The uncinated lateral border is attached to the frontal process of the maxilla while its free edge lies medially. Its breath, length, and thickness vary from one to another. The uncinated is attached to the maxillary process superiorly, which curves laterally. The inferior process arises from the inferior edge being in contact with the inferior turbinate.

There are several attachments of the uncinate process. Although there are several others, the three main variations in attachments are [15].

1. **Lamina papyracea.** Attachment to the lamina papyracea allows the frontal sinus to drain just medial to the uncinated into the middle meatus, while the area between the uncinate and lamina papyracea forms the recess terminalis, which is a blind recess.

2. **Lateral aspect of the middle turbinate**. Its attachment allows the frontal sinus to drain medially and directly into the ethmoidal infundibulum

3. **Skull base**. Frontal sinus drainage is similar to 2 above.

Other anatomical variations of the uncinate process are described.

4.2 Pneumatized uncinate

The pneumatized or aeration of the uncinate process also known as a bulla may obstruct the OMC and result in diseases of the paranasal sinuses (**Figure 9**). It is

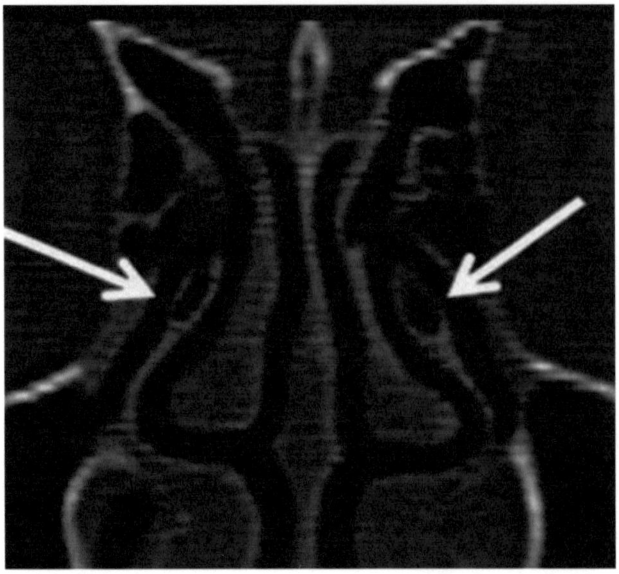

Figure 9.
Bilateral aeration of uncinate process.

believed that the uncinate bulla may be a continuation of the agar nasi (anterior most ethmoidal air cell) from above [16]. It should not be mistaken with a Haler cell of the maxillary sinus.

4.3 Bifid uncinate

A bifid uncinate has two superior bony projections, its significance unknown and rare (**Figure 10**) [16].

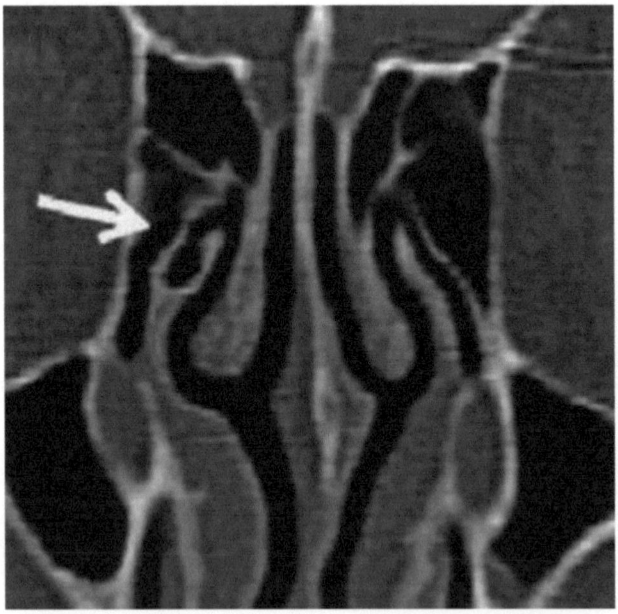

Figure 10.
A bifid right uncinate process.

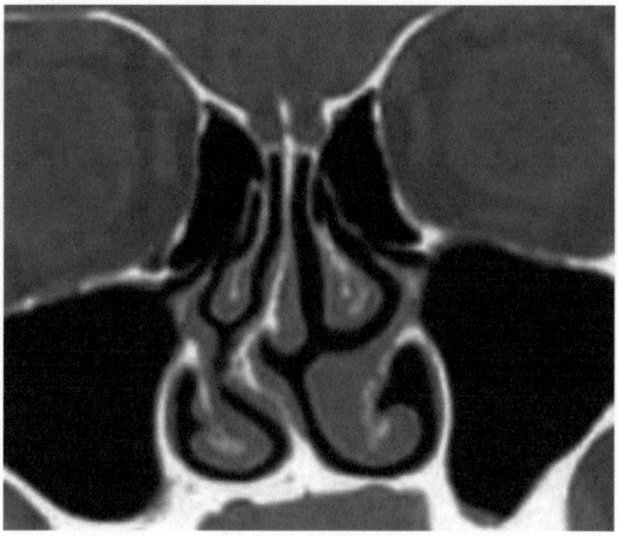

Figure 11.
A curved uncinate process.

4.4 Curved uncinate

A curved uncinate can either be located horizontally or vertically (**Figure 11**). A horizontally located uncinate is often seen together with a large bulla ethmoidalis. It may curve medially to form a Kaufmann's double middle turbinate [16, 17].

4.5 Atelectatic uncinate

An atelectatic uncinate is one that is not developed and hypoplastic and may be adherent to the medial wall of the orbit or lamina papyracea. It should be identified radiologically to avoid violation to the lamina papyracea. Otherwise, one may assume the lamina papyracea is the uncinate process and attempt to remove it resulting in orbital complications. It is associated with maxillary sinus hypoplasia or silent sinus syndrome [16].

5. Olfactory fossa

The olfactory fossa is a depression of the anterior cranial cavity formed by the cribriform plate, thus discontinuing the nasal cavity beneath from the cranial fossa above. The crista galli forms the medial boundary and lateral lamella of the cribriform forms the lateral boundary. The lateral lamella is the thinnest bone and may be dehiscent. The olfactory fossa contains olfactory nerves. A three-tier classification of the depth of the olfactory fossa was performed by Keros on 450 samples (**Figure 12**). It should be measured at the coronal view [18]. Beware of asymmetry within the right and left.

Keros Type 1.

Depth of OF is 1–3 mm. The cribriform is almost in level with the roof of the ethmoid. Eyeballing a coronal section of the CT scan, the cribriform is often above an imaginary horizontal line connecting the center of both eyeballs. It is the second most common variation.

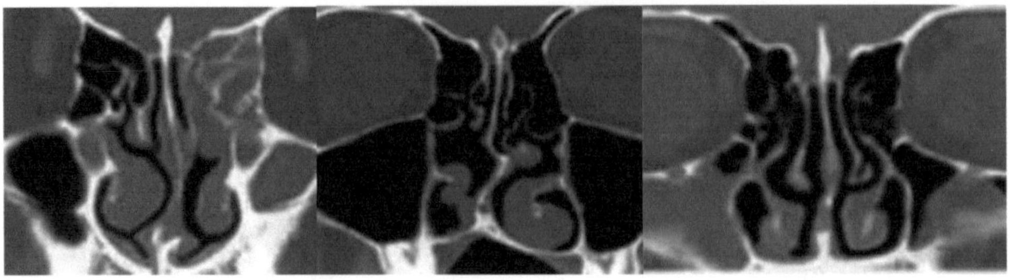

Figure 12.
Coronal view of the CT of the paranasal sinuses demonstrating a) Keros type 1, b) Keros type 2, and c) Keros type 3.

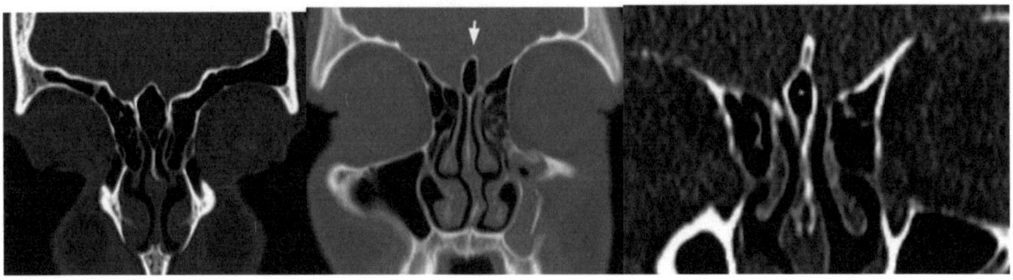

Figure 13.
Pneumatization of crista galli from left a) small; b) moderate, and c) large.

Keros Type 2.

Depth of OF is 4–7 mm. The cribriform is lower than that of type 1 resulting in a higher vertical length of the lateral lamella. Eyeballing a coronal section of the CT scan, the cribriform is just above the imaginary horizontal line connecting the centers of both eyeballs. It is the most common variation.

Keros Type 3.

Depth of OF is 8–16 mm. The cribriform is even lower than 1 and 2 with an even higher vertical length of the lateral lamella predisposing to greater risk of penetration if the surgeon is not careful during an endoscopic sinus surgery. This may lead to CSF leaks, meningocele, encephalocele, bleeding, and meningitis. It has been termed as the dangerous ethmoid. Eyeballing the coronal section of the CT scan, the cribriform is approximately at the level of the imaginary horizontal line joining the center of both eyeballs. It is the least common variation.

6. Crista galli

Crista galli is the outpouching of the ethmoid bone into the anterior cranial fossa. It sits in the center and divides the olfactory bulbs into the right and left. A pneumatized crista galli (**Figure 13a–c**) is thought to be caused by extension of aeration from the ethmoid bones and classified as small, moderate or large. However, there is strong evidence that pneumatization of the frontal sinus instead may extend into the crista galli [19]. Its incidence is less than 5%. The pneumatization can be surrounded by bony walls or spongy bones, which has been associated with chronic inflammation of the sinuses and in rare cases, a mucocele within [20].

7. Frontal sinus

The frontal sinus is the only sinus not present at birth. Pneumatization starts at the age 2 and reaches the orbital roof by age 5 to 7 years and attains adult size by 12 years.

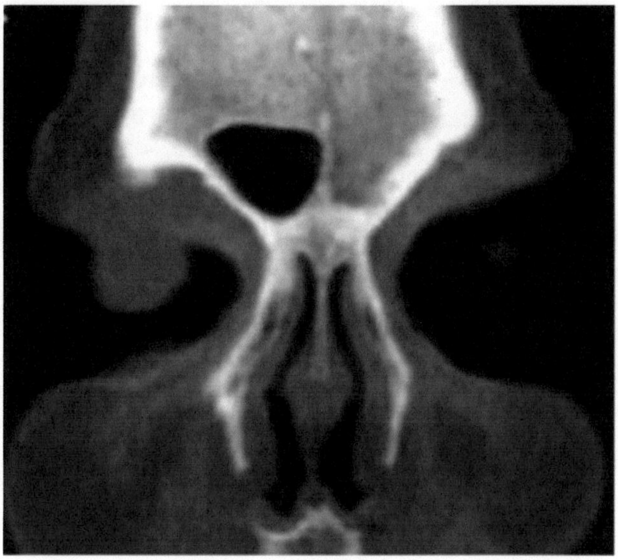

Figure 14.
Serial view of coronal CT scan paranasal sinuses showing asymmetry of the frontal sinuses with a rudimentary left frontal sinus.

The frontal sinus comprises two sinuses extending in the squamous part of the temporal bone and is separated by bony septum. Since each separated sinus (right and left) develops independently, they are expected to be asymmetrically pneumatized (**Figure 14**). Most commonly the larger sinus passes over the midline and overlaps the other [3].

The anterior and posterior walls of the sinuses are called the outer and inner tables. Unlike the thick bony wall of the outer table, the relatively thin inner table bony plate separates the frontal sinus from the cranial fossa posteriorly. The foramina of Breschet that consists of venous drainage channels is found on the inner table of the sinus and is the source of infection spread from the sinus intracranially. These foramina are sites of mucosal invagination within the bone, and the outcome of incomplete mucosal removal from these sites during sinus obliteration procedure predisposes to the development of mucocele.

Frontal sinus ostium is located at the posteromedial portion of the sinus's floor. The narrowest path of the frontal sinus drainage pathway (an hourglass shape) corresponds to the frontal beak, which represents the frontal sinus ostium. Anatomically, the frontal sinus lies superior to the beak and the frontal recess inferior to the beak. The size and patency of the frontal sinus ostium is determined by the thickness of the frontal beak (frontonasal process of maxilla).

A large agger nasi cell results in a small frontal beak and a wider frontal sinus ostium. On the contrary, a small agger nasi cell results in a prominent frontal beak and a narrow ostium. A larger agger nasi cell may compromise the frontal sinus drainage pathway at the level of the frontal recess inferiorly.

7.1 Hypoplastic frontal sinus

Hypoplastic frontal sinus is found in 4% and aplasia in 5% of the population [21].

7.2 Frontoethmoidal cell

Frontal sinuses may contain air cells as projections from the ethmoidal sinus. The modified Wormald classification of the frontoethmoidal cell (frontal cells) classifies them into several types [22].

Type 1 frontal cell—single frontal recess cell above agger nasi cell but below frontal ostium (**Figure 15**).

Type 2 frontal cells—two or more frontal recess cells above agger nasi cell but below frontal ostium (**Figure 16**).

Type 3 frontal cell—single cell above the agger nasi with extension into the frontal sinus through the frontal ostium but not exceeding 50% vertical height of the ipsilateral frontal sinus (**Figure 17**).

Type 4 frontal cell—either single cell above the agger nasi with extension into the frontal sinus through the frontal ostium and exceeding 50% vertical height of the ipsilateral frontal sinus or an isolated cell within the frontal sinus (**Figure 18**).

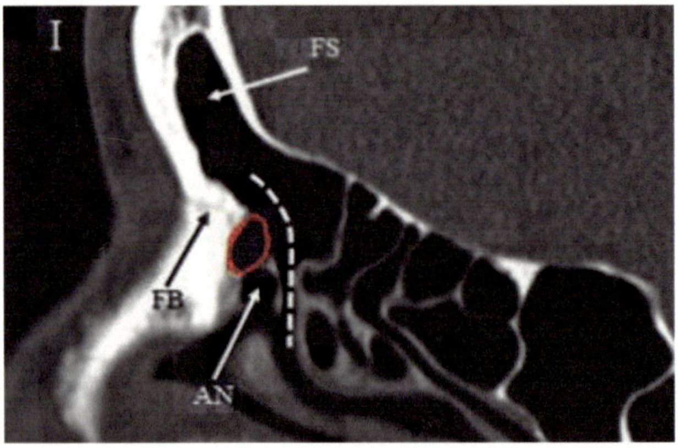

Figure 15.
Parasagittal view demonstrating type 1 frontal cell in red, FS (frontal cell), FB (frontal beak corresponding to frontal ostium), AN (agger nasi cell), white-dashed line represents the midway of the frontal sinus vertical line.

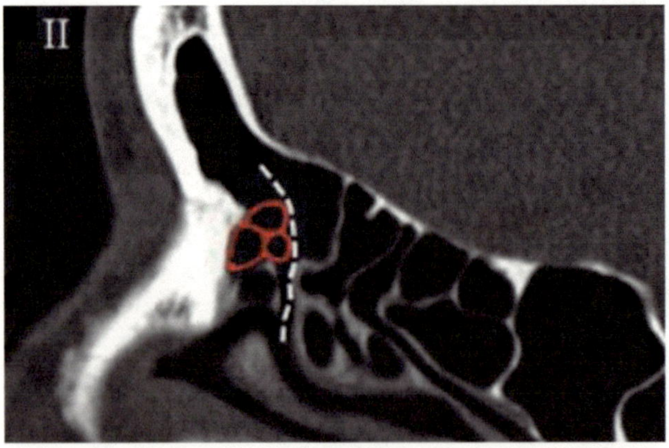

Figure 16.
Parasagittal view demonstrating type 2 frontal cells in red, white-dashed line represents the midway of the frontal sinus vertical line.

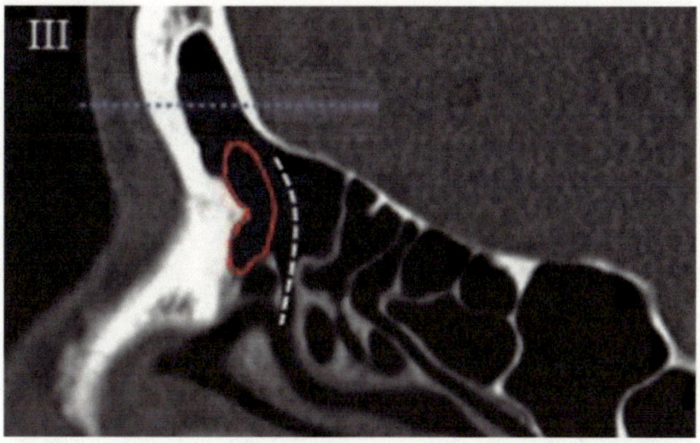

Figure 17.
Parasagittal view demonstrating type 3 frontal cell in red, white-dashed line represents the midway of the frontal sinus vertical line.

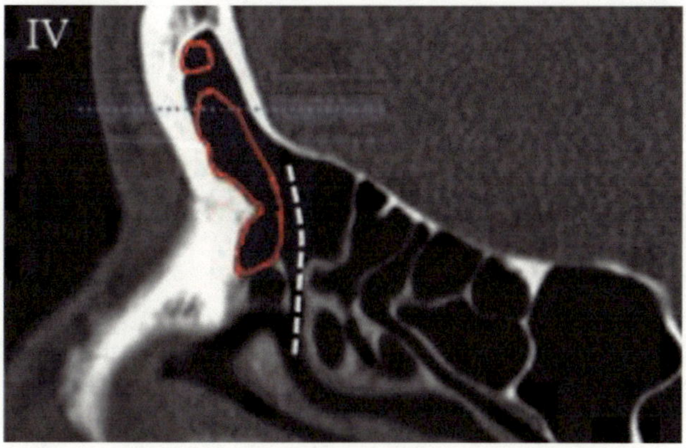

Figure 18.
Parasagittal view demonstrating type 4 frontal cell in red, white-dashed line represents the midway of the frontal sinus vertical line.

7.3 Frontal bullar cell

It consists of a single cell that extends from suprabullar region into frontal sinus superiorly along the posterior wall of frontal recess This is unlike the suprabullar cell that does not extend into the frontal sinus. Its anterior wall is related to frontal sinus and its posterior to anterior cranial fossa. One should be cautious during surgery while opening this cell, not to cause unintentional trauma to anterior skull base.

7.4 Frontal intersinus septal cell

This occurs when an intersinus septum is pneumatized and may communicate with either one of the frontal sinuses or could be completely an isolated air cell, which may compromise the frontal sinus ostium patency (**Figure 19**).

8. Maxillary sinus and natural ostium

The maxillary sinus is present at birth. By 12 weeks *in utero*, the ethmoid maxillary recess projects out pouches laterally to form the maxillary sinus. At 3 months, ventrodorsal dimensions are 2.5 mm and by birth it is 7 mm [23].

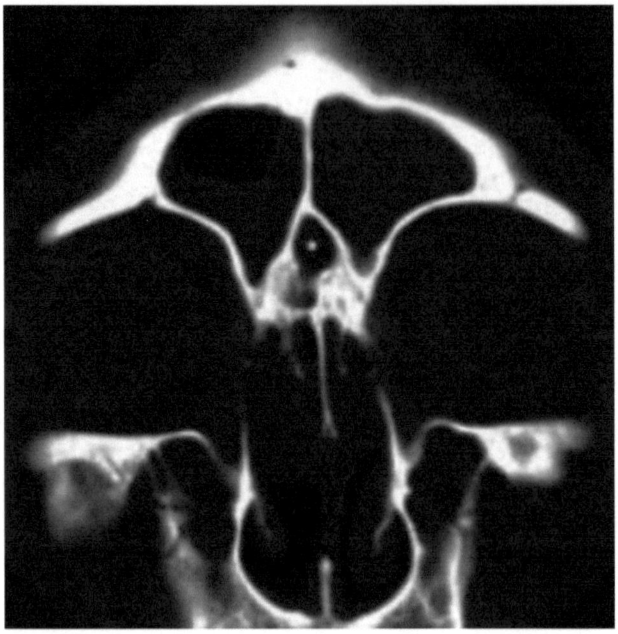

Figure 19.
Serial view of coronal CT scan paranasal sinuses showing a frontal intersinus septum (asterisk).

8.1 Agenesis/hypoplasia

Although maxillary sinus hypoplasia and agenesis is common, it is often asymptomatic and identified incidentally on imaging (**Figure 20**). It may be unilateral or bilateral. In higher grades of hypoplasia, the uncinate follows suit and it becomes more difficult to identify the natural ostia. Postulations of hypoplasia include congenital failure of development, chronic infection halting growth, and failure of

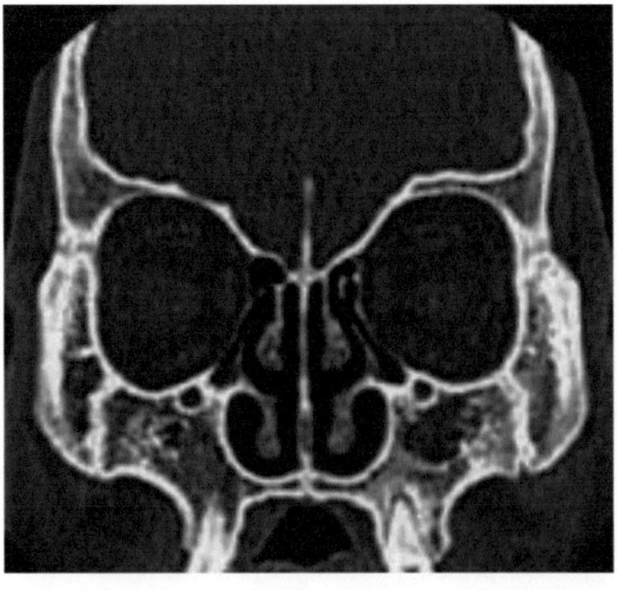

Figure 20.
Serial view of coronal CT scan of paranasal sinuses showing agenesis of the maxillary sinuses.

development of the uncinate process affecting that of the maxillary sinus [22]. Therefore, hypoplasia of the maxillary sinus can be classified into three [23]:

I. Normal uncinate and infundibular process with mild sinus hypoplasia and mucosal thickening,

II. Hypoplastic or absent uncinate and infundibular process with significant sinus hypoplasia and total opacification of sinus,

III. Absent uncinate process with profound hypoplasia and shallow cleft at lateral nasal wall.

Therefore, preoperative identification of hypoplasia and poorly developed uncinate processes is crucial to prevent iatrogenic trauma to the lamina papyracea.

8.2 Silent sinus syndrome

Although a syndrome, silent sinus syndrome (SSS) may cause an anatomical abnormality to the maxillary sinus. It is a phenomenon whereby a normally developed maxillary sinus is reabsorbed. This is believed to be due to chronic maxillary sinusitis atelectasis whereby the absence of ventilation causes the sinus to reabsorbed over time. It is believed that a large fluffy uncinate acts as a one-way air outflow valve mechanism within the OMC resulting in maxillary atelectasis [24]. The orbital floor will bow into the maxillary sinus often entrapping orbital muscles resulting in enophthalmos, sunken orbital sulci, and double vision in a previously normal individual. There may or may not be a history of rhinosinusitis symptoms. Unlike a maxillary sinuses agenesis or hypoplasia, SSS is not congenial and is acquired resulting in progressive changes over months in an individual with a normally developed maxillary sinus prior. Besides that, its criteria include no major nasal pathology, previous trauma, and with no previous congenital deformity [24]. Imaging in confirmatory and treatment involves a FESS with considerations of orbital floor reconstruction.

8.3 Intersinus septa

The maxillary intersinus septum may occur in 21.6 to 66.7% of patients (**Figure 21**). Many have tried to classify it based on its location in relation to the premolars and molars. It may obstruct mucosa flow and result in sinusitis. It is

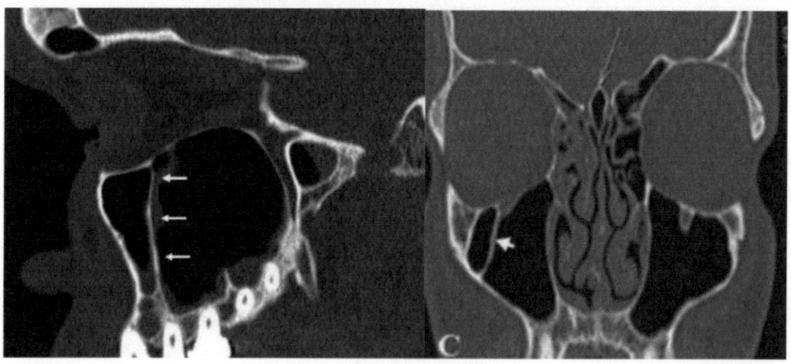

Figure 21.
Serial views of sagittal and coronal CT scan of paranasal sinuses showing right intersinus maxillary septa.

considered if it is more than 2.5 mm in height. It is said to be more common in adentulous patients [25].

8.4 Accessory ostium

An accessory ostium is one which is located away from the hiatus semilunaris. It occurs in less than 20% of individuals. Accessory ostium is more frequently located within the posterior fontanelle but existence within the anterior fontanelle is possible. It is often less than 1.5 mm in diameter. In a virgin nose, an encounter of a maxillary ostium within the posterior fontanelle is most likely an accessory ostium. The presence of an accessory ostium may cause looping of air within the natural and accessory ostium resulting in recirculation syndrome whereby the patient develops maxillary sinusitis due to inadequate ventilation of the maxillary sinus. In such instances, the surgeon should make a communication between the natural and accessory ostium to form a common cavity during a middle meatal antrostomy [3, 23].

8.5 Haler cell (infraorbital cell)

A Haler cell is an anterior inferior projection of an ethmoidal air toward the underside of the orbit. It may cause obstruction of the infundibulum and ventilation of the maxillary sinus (**Figure 22**).

9. Infraorbital nerve

The infraorbital nerve or V2 is the terminal branch of the maxillary division of the trigeminal nerve. It often runs within the infraorbital foramen, situated inferior to the infraorbital rim, and supplies the sensation of the cheek. Its course within the infraorbital foramen from the orbit to the cheek may vary (**Figure 23**). It is often at risk during a Caldwell-Luc procedure. Ference et al. 2015 have classified the variations into three [26]:

Type 1: Nerve within the sinus roof,

Type 2: Nerve just below the roof and juxtaposed to it,

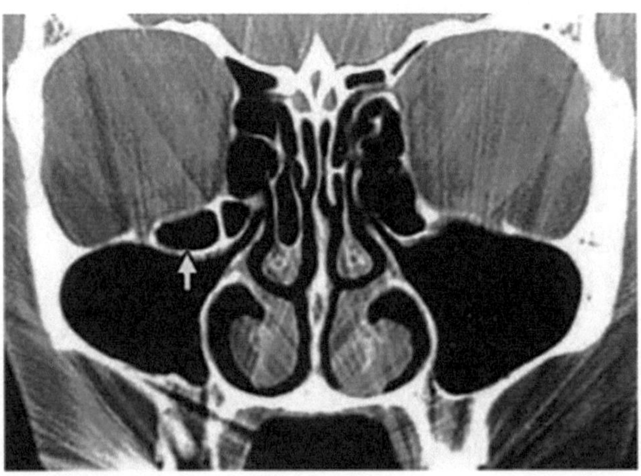

Figure 22.
A coronal CT scan of paranasal sinuses showing a right infraorbital cell.

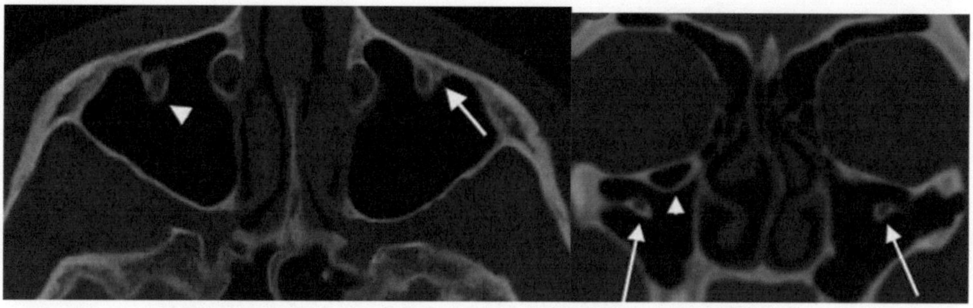

Figure 23.
Serial view of axial and coronal CT paranasal sinuses showing infraorbital nerve variations.

Type 3: Nerve descended into the sinus lumen, suspended within a septation of an infraorbital ethmoid cell.

Type 3 constitutes approximately 12.5% of the population with an 8.6 mm average below the roof of the maxillary sinus [26]. Preoperative identification of its dehiscent course from the maxillary sinus roof should be identified, and if maxillary sinus surgery is performed, its identification during surgery is crucial for preservation. Although endoscopic sinus surgery poses less risk, care should be taken when stripping of the maxillary sinus mucosa in cases of benign tumors such as inverted papilloma and breaking of septations of the maxillary sinus. It may also be damaged during trauma to the midface or cheek. Trauma to the infraorbital nerve may cause paresthesia to the region of the ipsilateral cheek.

10. Ethmoidal sinus

The anterior ethmoidal sinus is present at birth, while the posterior is initially fluid filled and continues to develop until the age of 12 [27]. It is formed by the ethmoidal bone forming multiple pyramidal air cells. It is bounded laterally by the eyes, which is being separated from the nasal cavity by the thin lamina papyrecea. Posteriorly is the face of the sphenoid, and anterior is the agar nasi cell. With reference to the base of skull, the axilla of the middle turbinate divides the base of skull to the cribriform plate medial to it and fovea ethmoidalis (roof of ethmoid) lateral to it. Hence, the medial borders of the ethmoidal sinus bilaterally are the axilla of the middle turbinate [27]. It is important to appreciate that the skull base slopes inferiorly from the anterior to posterior direction. The basal lamella of the middle turbinate forms the separation between the anterior and posterior ethmoidal air cells. The anterior ethmoids have smaller and greater number of air cells compared with the posterior. The anterior ethmoidal air cells drain into the osteomeatal complex, while the posterior ethmoidal air cells drain into the sphenoethmoidal recess posteriorly.

10.1 Ethmoid bulla

The degree of pneumatization of the ethmoidal bulla may vary, with failure to pneumatized in 8% population (torus ethmoidalis or totus lateralis) [7]. On the contrary, a giant bulla fills out the entire middle meatus encroaching the space between the uncinate process and the middle turbinate, with lamina papyracea forming its lateral relationship. The ethmoidal bulla may fuse superiorly with the skull base forming the posterior wall of frontal recess, failing which a small

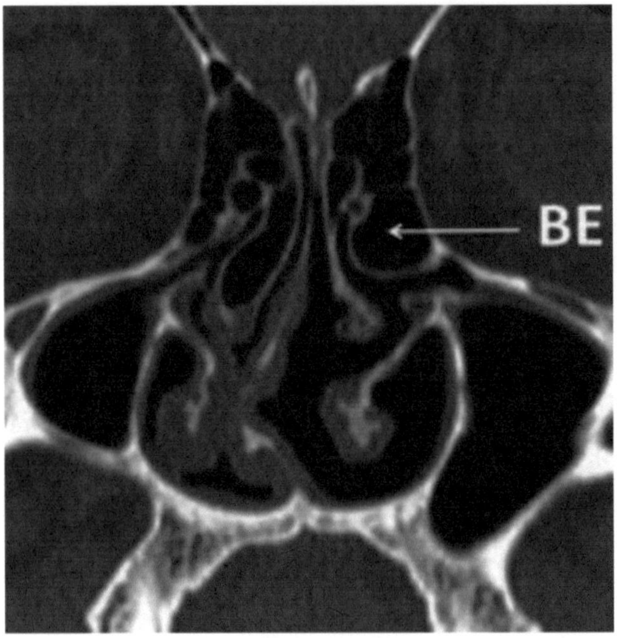

Figure 24.
Serial coronal view of the paranasal sinuses showing a prominent left bulla ethmoidalis (BE).

suprabullar recess may connect anteriorly to the frontal recess. Posteriorly, it may fuse with the ground lamella over a variable length. The ethmoidal bulla is superior to the ethmoidal infundibulum on coronal CT images (**Figure 24**).

10.2 Anterior ethmoidal artery

The anterior ethmoidal artery, a branch of the ophthalmic artery, crosses the orbit, the ethmoid labyrinth, and the anterior fossa of the skull. It enters the olfactory fossa through the lateral lamella of the cribriform plate (anterior ethmoidal sulcus),

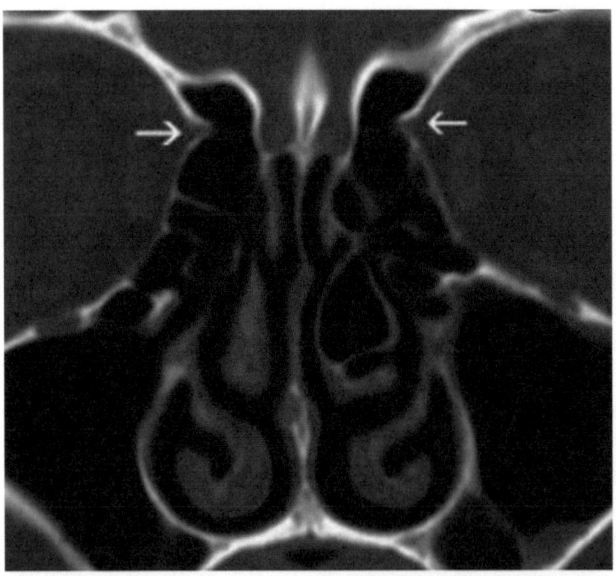

Figure 25.
Serial coronal view of the paranasal sinuses showing bilateral anterior ethmoidal artery notch (arrows).

where the bone is extremely thin and at highest risk in nasal endoscopic surgery (**Figure 25**). The course of the anterior ethmoidal artery is relatively variable in the ethmoidal roof and is vulnerable to injury during surgical procedures.

11. Lamina papyracea

The lamina papyracea is the thin bone that forms the medial wall of the orbit and lateral wall of the ethmoidal sinus. It is also known as the orbital lamina of the ethmoidal bone. Dehiscence of the lamina papyracea may occur and can be as a result of trauma, infection, or tumor. Its dehiscence may be small or may extend posteriorly to the basal lamella. Some may contain infraorbital fat, while some contain mucosa of the ethmoidal sinus. Chronic nasal polyposis may exert pressure to the thin bone and weaken it resulting in dehiscence and protuberance of orbital content. Its protuberance may cause invagination of periorbita with or without the medial rectus, which may mimic ethmoiditis (**Figure 26a** and **b**). Its presence is of concern especially during endoscopic sinus surgery where injury to the periorbita and the medial rectus may occur [28].

12. Sphenoid sinus

The vomer usually joins the sphenoid sinus in the midline, and this is a very reliable surgical landmark. The sphenoid sinus occupies the body of the sphenoid. Anatomically, there are two asymmetrical sinuses separated off-midline by intersphenoid bony septum. The sphenoid sinus drains into the sphenoethmoidal recess through the solitary sphenoid ostium located in the anterior wall of the sinus, which opens medially to superior turbinate. The ostium is located more medially toward the rostrum, about 10 to 12 mm superior to the upper border of the choana, and about 7 cm from anterior nasal spine at an angle of 30 degree to the nasal floor The ostium is ideally superomedial to the tail of the superior turbinate. The posterior septal artery crosses the sphenoid face from the lateral nasal wall to the posterior end of the nasal septum. In 65% of cases, it bifurcates into the superior or inferior branches before crossing, and in 35% cases, it bifurcates after crossing, inferior to the ostium. The posterior septal artery is about 5 mm below the ostium. On widening the ostium, it is safer to widen it horizontally and superiorly.

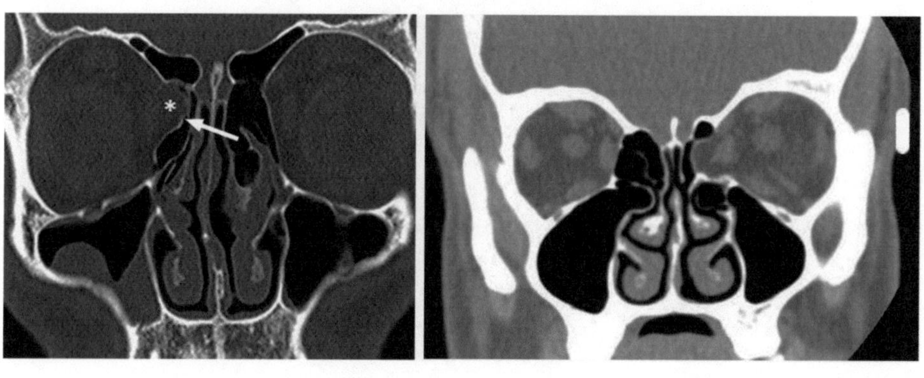

Figure 26.
A serial coronal CT scan of the paranasal sinuses showing a) a right extraconal fat protrusion into the anterior ethmoidal sinus (arrow) and B) a left periorbital fat and medial rectus protrusion into the anterior ethmoidal sinus.

The vital structures surrounding the sphenoid sinus are the pituitary gland, optic nerves, cavernous sinuses and carotid arteries, maxillary divisions (V2) of trigeminal nerves within the foramen rotundum, and vidian canals. These structures are easily seen as indentations on the sinus's roof and walls internally, which are related to the degree of pneumatization of the sinus.

Posterior to the sinus lie the pons and the posterior cranial fossa and the roof is related to the pituitary gland and middle cranial fossa. On the posterior wall of the sinus bilaterally, the optic nerve crosses the border formed by the roof and the lateral wall. The cavernous segment of the internal carotid canals can be seen as bony prominences on the posterolateral walls of the sinus. The maxillary division of trigeminal nerves passes through the foramina rotunda toward the pterygopalatine fossa bilaterally within the lateral sphenoid walls. Within the vidian or pterygoid canals, the vidian nerve crosses the lateral sides of the sinus floor.

12.1 Agenesis or hypoplasia

Sphenoid sinus agenesis (**Figure 27**) is a rare entity and usually associated with syndromes such as craniosynostosis, osteodysplasia, Down Syndrome, and Hand-Schuler-Christain Disease [29].

12.2 Pneumatization of sphenoid sinus

Depending on the degree of pneumatization, the sphenoid sinus is classified into three types as illustrated in the figures below:

1. Conchal: Sphenoid sinus agenesis or the conchal type occurs in a non-pneumatized sinus (0.7%) and is a relative contraindication for endoscopic trans-sphenoid skull base approach (**Figure 28**)

2. Presellar (**Figure 29**)

3. Sellar (**Figure 30**)

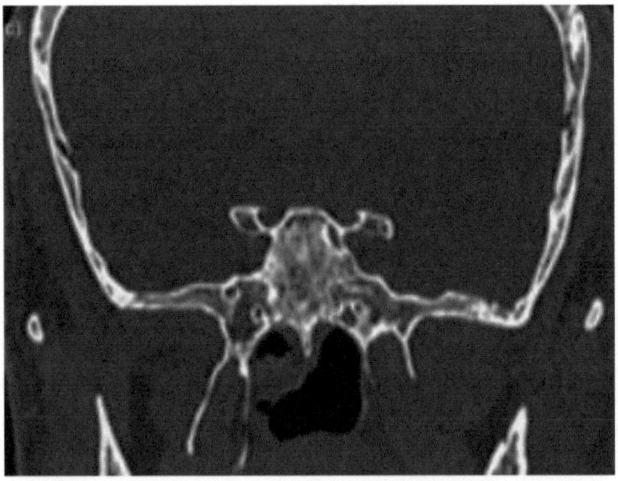

Figure 27.
Left periorbital fat and medial rectus protrusion into the anterior ethmoidal sinus.

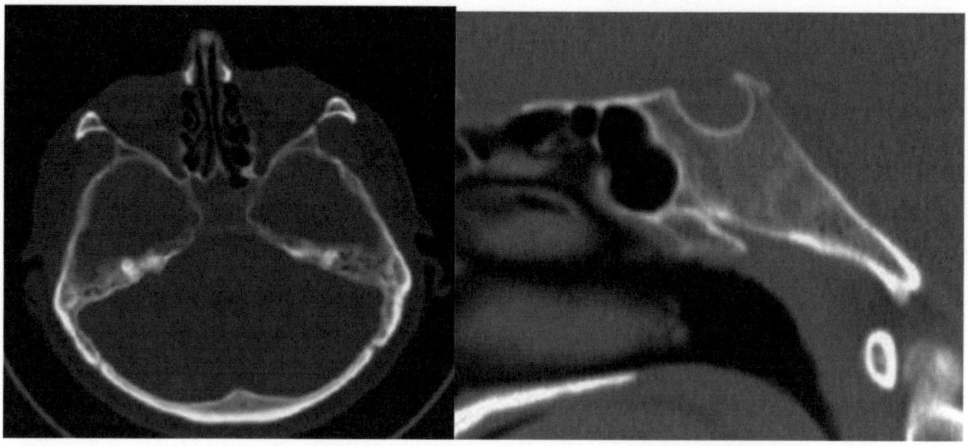

Figure 28.
Conchal type: A serial axial and coronal CT scan paranasal sinus showing the degree of pneumatization is limited to the anterior portion of the sphenoid body and not reaching the level of the anterior wall of Sella turcica (1–4%).

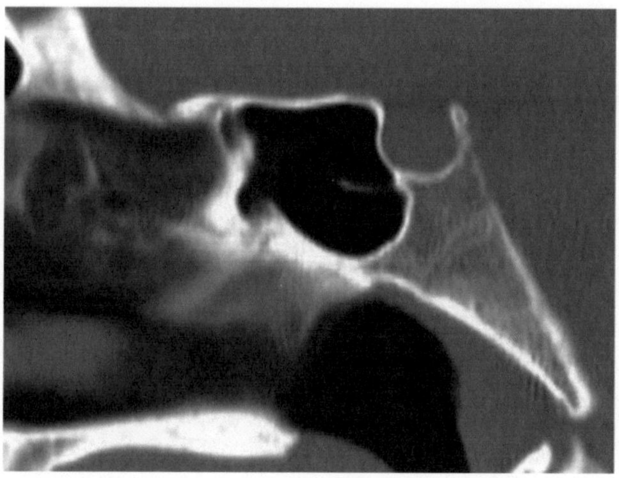

Figure 29.
Presellar type: A serial sagittal CT scan paranasal sinus showing pneumatization, which extends up to the vertical level of the anterior wall of the Sella turcica but not beyond it (35–40%).

12.3 Optic nerve dehiscence

Optic nerve canal dehiscence occurs in 4% cases where the bony canal is having a focal dehiscence and only sinus mucosa with neural sheath is separating the nerve from the sinus (**Figure 31**). The thickness of the wall of the optic canal that separates it from the sinus is less than 0.5 mm in 78% of cases.

12.4 Internal carotid artery dehiscence

Internal carotid artery dehiscence occurs when the region of the medial side of the bony canal separating the sinus from the artery is defective, exposing the internal carotid artery at risk during the endoscopic sphenoid surgery with an incidence of 8 to 25% of this variant (**Figure 32**) [30].

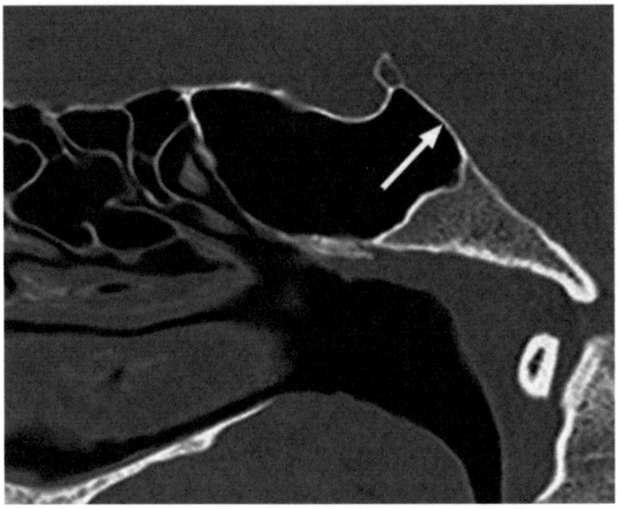

Figure 30.
Sella type: A serial sagittal view of paranasal sinuses showing pneumatization extending beyond the level of the anterior wall of the Sella turcica below the pituitary fossa and may reach posterior to the Sella turcica known as postsellar type (55–60%).

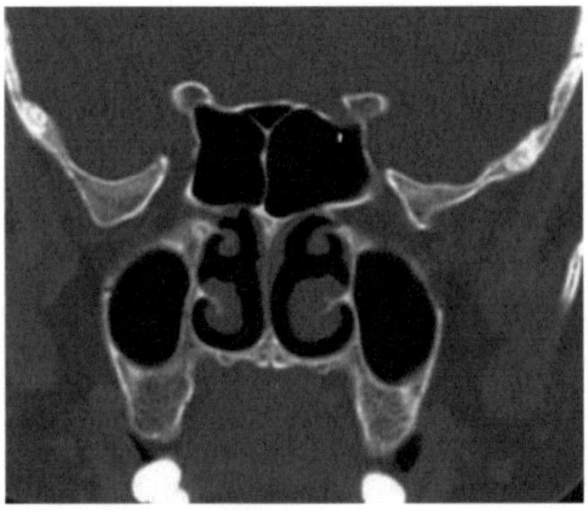

Figure 31.
A serial coronal view of paranasal sinuses showing dehiscence involving the left optic nerve cana (arrow).

12.5 Sphenoid sinus septation

The inter-sinus sphenoid septum may deviate off the midline and has an insertion into the internal carotid artery bony canal (**Figure 33**) or the optic canal. To avoid avulsion of the bony wall, excessive traction on the septum should be avoided in these cases especially in endoscopic pituitary surgery [31].

12.6 Sphenoid pneumatization

A pneumatized posterior nasal septum may occur from an extension of air from the sphenoid sinus or crista Galli, which rarely causes narrowing of the sphenoethmoidal region.

Supraoptic and infra-optic recess occurs in hyperpneumatized sphenoid sinus when pneumatization reaches superiorly (**Figure 34**) and inferiorly to the optic canal, resulting in these two recesses, respectively. The infra-optic recess or the opticocarotid recess lies between the optic canal and the internal carotid artery.

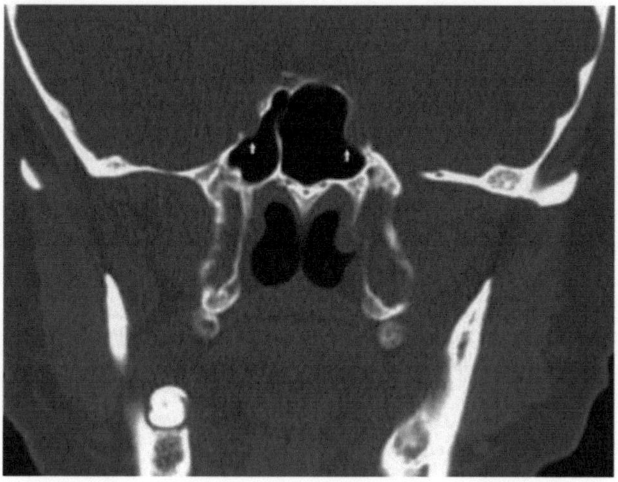

Figure 32.
A serial coronal view of paranasal sinuses showing dehiscence of bilateral internal carotid artery (arrows).

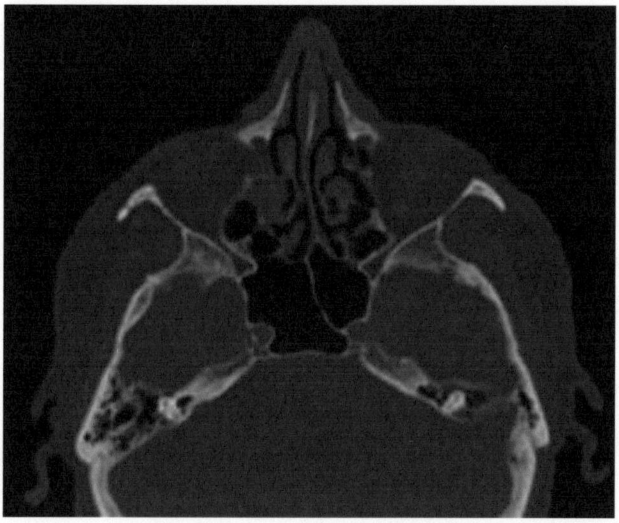

Figure 33.
A serial axial view of paranasal sinuses showing insertion of the inter-sinus septum into the left internal carotid artery bony canal.

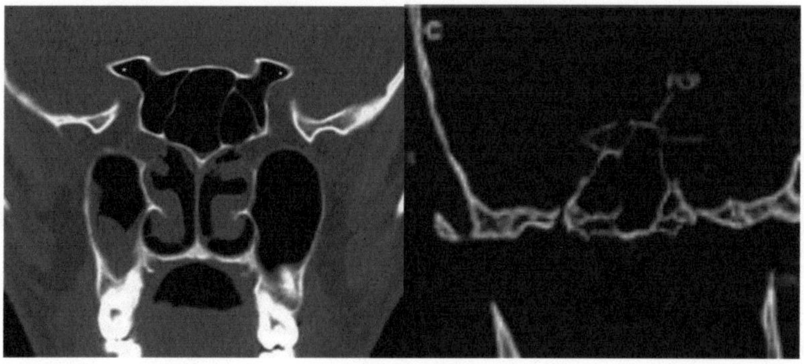

Figure 34.
Serial coronal views of paranasal sinuses showing bilateral pneumatization of anterior clinoid process (arrows) and posterior clinoid process (red arrow).

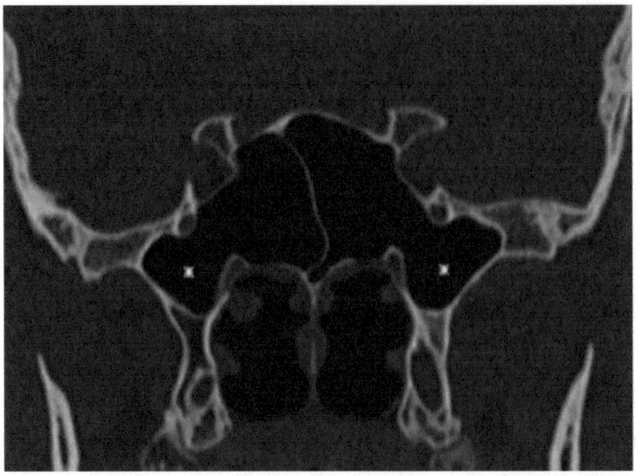

Figure 35.
A serial coronal view of paranasal sinuses showing extensive pneumatization between the maxillary (V2) and the vidian nerve resulting in pneumatized pterygoids (arrows).

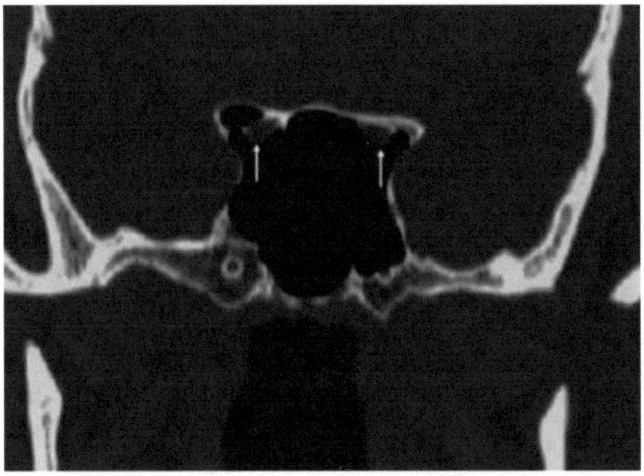

Figure 36.
Coronal view of paranasal sinuses showing bilateral Onodi cells (arrows).

Furthermore, the pneumatization may extend from the infra-optic recess to the anterior clinoid process.

Lateral recess occurs when pneumatization extends extensively inferolaterally between the maxillary (V2) and the vidian nerve (**Figure 35**).

12.7 Posterior ethmoid air cell

This is also known as Onodi cell, which refers to the extension of the posterior most ethmoidal cells superolateral to the sphenoid sinus into the anterior clinoid process (**Figure 36**). If they become infected or due to poor judgment by endoscopic surgeon, it can lead to injury to the optic canal.

13. Conclusion

The advent of CT scans and FESS has made the sinuses and its paranasal sinuses less of a mystery to us. More anatomical variations, its formation and functions will be discovered with time. Due to the presence of variations and its relationship to the orbit, skull base, neurological and vascular structures, a preoperative CT of the paranasal sinuses is vital for its identification and to prevent iatrogenic injuries. Coupled with the endoscopic findings, identification of anatomical variations may also give clues to the cause, appropriate identification, and treatment to the symptoms and pathology (such as sinus infection) faced by the patients.

Author details

Hardip Singh Gendeh[1] and Balwant Singh Gendeh[1,2]*

1 Department of Otorhinolaryngology, Head and Neck Surgery, Universiti Kebangsaan Malaysia Medical Center, Kuala Lumpur, Malaysia

2 Pantai Hospital Kuala Lumpur, Kuala Lumpur, Malaysia

*Address all correspondence to: bsgendeh@gmail.com

References

[1] Kane KJ. The early history and development of functional endoscopic sinus surgery. The Journal of Laryngology and Otology. 2020;**134**(1): 8-13

[2] Messerklinger W. Technique and possibilities of nasal endoscopy [in German]. HNO. 1972;**20**:133-135

[3] Gendeh BS. Endoscopic Sinus Surgery: State of the Art Technique. Bangi: Universiti Kebangsaan Malaysia Publication; 2004

[4] Dhingra PL, Dhingra S. Diseases of Ear, Nose and Throat & Head and Neck Surgery. 7th ed. India: RELX India Pvt. Ltd.; 2018

[5] Bolger WE, Butzin CA, Parsons DS. Paranasal sinus bony anatomic variations and mucosal abnormalities: CT analysis for endoscopic sinus surgery. The Laryngoscope. 1991; **101**(1):56-64

[6] O'Brien WT Sr, Hamelin S, Weitzel EK. The preoperative sinus CT: Avoiding a "CLOSE" call with surgical complications. Radiology. 2016;**281**(1): 10-21

[7] Alsaied AS. Paranasal sinus anatomy: What the surgeon needs to know. In: Gendeh BS, editor. Paranasal Sinuses. Intect: Croatia; 2017

[8] Arslan H, Aydınlıoğlu A, Bozkurt M, Egeli E. Anatomic variations of the paranasal sinuses: CT examination for endoscopic sinus surgery. Auris, Nasus, Larynx. 1999;**26**(1):39-48

[9] Gray LP. Deviated nasal septum. Incidence and etiology. The Annals of Otology, Rhinology & Laryngology. Supplement. 1978;**87**(50):3-20

[10] Shpilberg KA, Daniel SC, Doshi AH, Lawson W, Som PM. CT of anatomic variants of the paranasal sinuses and nasal cavity: Poor correlation with radiologically significant rhinosinusitis but importance in surgical planning. AJR. American Journal of Roentgenology. 2015;**204**(6):1255-1260

[11] Gendeh BS, Tan VES. Open septorhinoplasty: Operative technique and grafts. The Medical Journal of Malaysia. 2006;**62**(1):13-18

[12] Yenigun A, Ozturan O, Buyuk PN. Pneumatized septal turbinate. Auris, Nasus, Larynx. 2014;**41**(3):310-312

[13] Azman M, Gendeh BS. Septal turbinates: An entity with physiological importance. Brunei International Medical Journal. 2011;**7**(3):168-172

[14] Stammberger H, Koop W, Dekornfeld TJ. Special endoscopic anatomy. In: Stammberger H, Hawke M, editors. Functional Endoscopic Sinus Surgery: The Messerklinger Technique. Philadelphia, PA: BC Decker; 1991. pp. 61-90

[15] Güngör G, Okur N, Okur E. Uncinate process variations and their relationship with ostiomeatal complex: A pictorial essay of multidetector computed tomography (MDCT) findings. Polish Journal of Radiology. 2016;**20**(81):173-180

[16] Cagici CA, Ozer C, Yilmaz I, Bolat FA, Cakmak O. Solitary polyps of the uncinate process. Ear, Nose, & Throat Journal. 2007;**86**(2):94-96

[17] Tan HM, Chong VFH. CT of the paranasal sinuses: Normal anatomy, variants and pathology. CME Radiology. 2001;**2**:120-125

[18] Keros P. On the practical value of differences in the level of the lamina cribrosa of the ethmoid. Zeitschrift fur

Laryngologie, Rhinologie, Otologie und Ihre Grenzgebiete. 1962;**41**:809-813

[19] Som PM, Park EE, Naidich TP, Lawson W. Crista galli pneumatization is an extension of the adjacent frontal sinuses. American Journal of Neuroradiology. 2009;**30**(1):31-33

[20] Mladina R, Antunović R, Cingi C, Muluk NB, Skitarelić N, Malić M. An anatomical study of pneumatized crista galli. Neurosurgical Review. 2017;**40**(4): 671-678

[21] Khanduri S, Singh N, Bhadury S, Ansari AA, Chaudhary M. Combined aplasia of frontal and sphenoid sinuses with hypoplasia of ethmoid and maxillary sinuses. Indian Journal of Otolanygology and Head & Neck Surgery. 2015;**67**(4):434-437

[22] Wormald PJ, Hoseman W, Callejas C, Weber RK, Kennedy DW, Citardi MJ, et al. The international frontal sinus anatomy classification (IFAC) and classification of the extent of endoscopic frontal sinus surgery (EFSS). International Forum Allergy & Rhinology. 2016;**6**(7): 677-696

[23] Bolger WE, Woodruff WW, Morehead J, Parsons DS. Maxillary sinus hypoplasia: Classification and description of associated uncinate process hypoplasia. Otolaryngology–Head and Neck Surgery. 1990;**103**(5): 759-765

[24] Bossolesi P, Autelitano L, Brusati R, Castelnuovo P. The silent sinus syndrome: Diagnosis and surgical treatment. Rhinology. 2008;**46**(4): 308-316

[25] Maestre-Ferrín L, Galán-Gil S, Rubio-Serrano M, Peñarrocha-Diago M, Peñarrocha-Oltra D. Maxillary sinus septa: A systematic review. Medicina Oral, Patología Oral y Cirugía Bucal. 2010;**15**(2):383-386

[26] Ference EH, Smith SS, Conley D, Chandra RK. Surgical anatomy and variations of the infraorbital nerve. The Laryngoscope. 2015;**125**(6):1296-1300

[27] Ogle OE, Weinstock RJ, Friedman E. Surgical anatomy of the nasal cavity and paranasal sinuses. Oral and Maxillofacial Surgery Clinics of North America. 2012; **24**(2):156-166

[28] Moulin G, Dessi P, Chagnaud C, Bartoli JM, Vignoli P, Gaubert JY, et al. Dehiscence of the lamina papyracea of the ethmoid bone: CT findings. AJNR. American Journal of Neuroradiology. 1994;**15**(1):151-153

[29] Anik I, Anik Y, Koc K, Ceylan S. Agenesis of sphenoid sinus. Clinical Anatomy. 2005;**18**(3):217-219. DOI: 10.1002/ca.20096

[30] Padhye V, Valentine R, Wormald PJ. Management of carotid artery injury in endonasal surgery. International Archives of Otorhinolaryngology. 2014;**18**(Suppl 2): S 173-S 178

[31] Lum SG, Gendeh BS, Husain S, Izaham A, Tan HJ, Gendeh HS. Internal carotid artery injury during endoscopic sinus surgery: Our experience and review of the literature. Acta Otorhinolaryngologica Italica. 2019; **39**(2):130-136

Section 2

Maxillofacial

Chapter 5

Sino-Nasal Changes Associated with Midfacial Expansion: An Overview

G. Dave Singh

Abstract

The concept of palatal expansion can be viewed as an anachronism since the delivery and scope of this clinical technique has changed dramatically over the past few decades. Indeed, since the palatal complex does not exist in isolation, clinicians ought to be cognizant of how palatal expansion affects contiguous midfacial structures. Because of this structural arrangement, surgical and non-surgical palatal expansion can have clinical consequences on the dentoalveolar structures, which are dependent on bony remodeling of the maxillo-palatine complex. In addition, it can also be suggested that morphologic alterations of the maxillary air sinus might lead to functional and clinical improvements of inflammatory changes associated with rhinosinusitis. Furthermore, enhancements in the nasal airway could affect a host of other conditions, including nasal breathing and obstructive sleep apnea, etc. Therefore, the aim of this chapter is to review the effects of midfacial expansion techniques on contiguous structures, including the paranasal sinuses.

Keywords: Maxillary sinus, nasal airway, sinusitis, palatal expansion, midfacial development

1. Introduction

The human air sinuses are enigmatic in that numerous functional attributes have been associated with them, including humidification, warming, and cleaning of inhaled air; biosynthesis, storage, and concentration of nitric oxide (NO); an anterior 'crumple zone' to withstand frontal trauma, and lightening of the skull, presumably for flight in extinct dinosaurs and extant birds. Recent evidence even goes on to suggest that the paranasal sinuses might be vestigial organs of breathing [1]. In any case, originally, clinical palatal expansion was pioneered as an orthodontic technique to widen the upper dental arch in attempt to improve jaw relations and/or tooth alignment. However, the maxillary air sinuses also lie above and lateral to the hard palate, while the dentoalveolar structures, such as the roots of the maxillary molars, can project into the sinus floor. Medially, the nasal airway communicates with the maxillary sinuses, including the ostio-meatal complex. Because of this diverse structural arrangement, non-surgical and surgical palatal expansion techniques might have clinical consequences on the maxillary air sinuses, which are dependent on bony remodeling and subsequent pneumatization of the maxillo-palatine complex. Therefore, an overview of various midfacial expansion procedures that might induce anatomic alterations of the maxillary air sinus, that may in turn lead to functional and clinical changes, is warranted.

2. Sinus changes associated with non-surgical midfacial expansion

Numerous studies have deployed 3D cone-beam computed tomography (CBCT) scans to quantify morphologic changes associated with rapid maxillary expansion (RME). For example, Lanteri et al. [2] evaluated midfacial changes after slow maxillary expansion and RME in 8 yr-old children. They found that the volumes of the nasal cavity and maxillary sinuses increased after treatment in both protocols. Conversely, Garrett et al. [3] had earlier reported that RME in 14 yr-olds was associated with an increase in nasal width but a decrease in maxillary sinus width, implying that the increase in nasal functional space was gained by displacing the maxillary air sinus volume, although clinical consequences of these changes were not noted. However, in a similar study on 13 yr-olds treated with banded and bonded maxillary expanders, Pangrazio-Kulbersh et al. [4] found that both appliances induced anterior and posterior skeletal widening of the hard palate via the midpalatal suture, and their study demonstrated increases in both nasal cavity volume and maxillary sinus volume. On the other hand, Almuzian et al. [5] provided further details of the RME approach in 13 yr-olds. Over a period of 2–3 weeks, an average palatal width-increase of 3.7 mm was noted in males and 2.8 mm in females. These linear changes were found to be correlated with maxillary sinus volume changes. Therefore, it can be surmised that anatomical differences in the outcome of RME might simply be explained by differences in the design, materials and protocols of the devices used.

A non-surgical variant of RME, maxillary protraction, deploys the use of facemasks (FM), particularly in cases of Class III malocclusion that exhibit a maxillary deficiency. Pamporakis et al. [6] assessed midfacial alterations, including the volume of the maxillary air sinuses in 10-yr-old children, associated with an RME-FM protocol for 10 days. Using this technique, they reported an overall increase in maxillary sinus volume post-treatment. However, the authors also noted that the RME-FM protocol did not affect all the maxillary sinuses, indicating that there may be a range of responses, presumably related to individual craniofacial morphology. In another variation of RME, alternate RME and constriction is sometimes deployed followed by FM. Onem-Ozbilen et al. [7] used this protocol on 10-yr-old children with a skeletal Class III phenotype, exhibiting maxillary retrognathia, over 10–12 months. It was found that the maxillary sinus volumes increased. Therefore, the authors concluded that different expansion devices and protocols can effect disparate changes in maxillary sinus volume. This deduction was borne out by the study of Erdur et al. [8] who used symmetric and asymmetric rapid maxillary expansion (ARME) treatments in patients aged 12-15 yrs. While maxillary sinus volume changes were greater in the RME group post-treatment, in the ARME group, no changes in sinus volume were found. Since bilateral symmetry is a feature of human development, these results are not perhaps surprising as the craniofacial system may regress to homeostasis once the devices are removed.

The age at which these various palatal expansion protocols are applied may also be pertinent. Most of these types of studies have been undertaken in pediatric populations but the efficacy of palatal expansion in older individuals is also worth considering. In fact, Machado-Júnior and Crespo [9] opine that maxillary expansion in adults requires further due diligence. In this regard, Kavand et al. [10] studied maxillary expansion with bone- and tooth-borne appliances in adolescents. They reported that both groups showed an increase in nasal cavity volume, but not maxillary sinus volume, even though the maxillary bone width increased. This is an interesting finding because by age 15 yrs. the second maxillary molars are often fully erupted and root formation is typically completed, giving little or no room for continued pneumatization until the maxillary third molars evacuate the body of the maxilla, which is rare, since unerupted, impacted wisdom teeth is a common finding on radiographs. Thus, in adolescents, RME is unlikely to result in an increase in maxillary sinus volume. In contrast, Singh and Kim [11] found that a biomimetic approach to palatal expansion increased maxillary sinus volume by some 6.5% in adults (mean age approx. 25 yrs.) accompanied by a mean palatal width increase of approx. 3 mm, which is similar to that achieved in teenagers as noted above. Therefore, while morphologic differences in the outcome of non-surgical RME might be explained by disparate designs, materials and protocols of the devices used, if the laws of biologic control, such as sutural homeostasis and pneumatization, are not violated, enhancement of maxillary sinus morphology might be possible even in adults, perhaps leading to improved clinical outcomes.

3. Functional sinus changes associated with non-surgical midfacial expansion

One of the roles of the paranasal sinuses is the biosynthesis of nitric oxide (NO). It is known that NO plays important roles in a diverse range of physiologic and patho-physiologic processes, including antimicrobial activity, pulmonary vascular resistance, alveolar oxygen transfer, neurotransmission, respiration, as well as its anti-inflammatory activities [12, 13]. Lundberg et al. [14] were some of the first to report that NO originates from the paranasal sinuses and that NO synthase is expressed in healthy sinus pneumocytes. In addition, Andersson et al. [15] found extremely high concentrations of NO in the paranasal sinuses, suggesting that the antra may act as NO reservoirs. Furthermore, Runer et al. [16] noted that NO is likely to be a regulator of mucociliary activity in the nasal airway. In contrast to these healthy states, Deja et al. [17] found significantly reduced NO production in maxillary sinuses of patients with sinusitis diagnosed using radiologic methods. Similarly, Naraghi et al. [18] reported that NO metabolites are higher in patients with chronic sinusitis and concluded that NO metabolites may play an important role in the pathogenesis of rhinosinusitis. In view of these findings, Degano et al. [19] investigated changes in NO concentration during the treatment of maxillary sinusitis. Using a protocol that included drainage, daily lavage, etc., a significant increase in the levels of maxillary and nasal NO was noted. Therefore, morphologic and functional optimization of the paranasal sinuses using non-surgical palatal expansion might be beneficial in the management of some sinus diseases.

In pediatric rhinitis, Wen et al. [20] consider that NO is a useful biomarker for both nasal inflammation and sinus ostial patency. In their study, they determined that obstruction of NO sino-nasal flow is likely associated with rhinosinusitis since NO concentrations returned to normal levels following antibiotic therapy. On the other hand, in a case series, Hwang et al. [21] reported their findings on pediatric rhinosinusitis during biomimetic oral appliance therapy (BOAT). **Figures 1a–3b** summarize their findings. In 3 consecutive pediatric patients (mean age 9 yrs.), Hwang et al. [21] used 3D cone-beam CT scans to show inflammatory maxillary sinus disease with circumferential mucosal thickening, obstructed ostio-meatuses, and enlarged inferior turbinates (**Figures 1a, 2a** and **3a**) prior to treatment. All 3 cases were treated using BOAT for approx. 10 months. Post-treatment, the sinuses were aerated without mucosal thickening; the sinus walls were intact, and the ostiomeatal units were patent (**Figures 1b, 2b** and **3b**). Although enhancement of maxillary air sinus structure

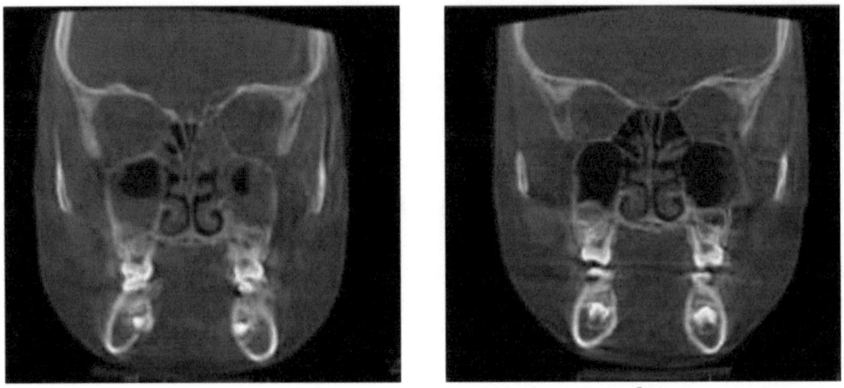

a b

Figure 1.
a: *Case 1: Pre-treatment nasal floor width is 17.7 mm;* ***b:*** *Post-treatment nasal floor width increased to 19.5 mm.*

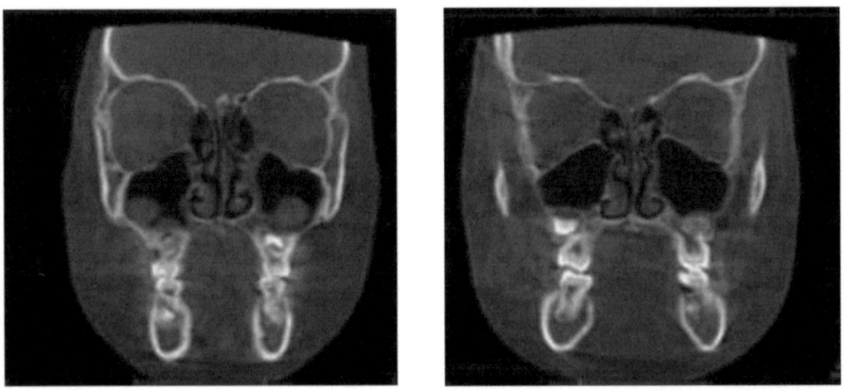

a b

Figure 2.
a: *Case 2: Pre-treatment nasal floor width is 17.6 mm;* ***b:*** *Post-treatment nasal floor width increased to 19.3 mm.*

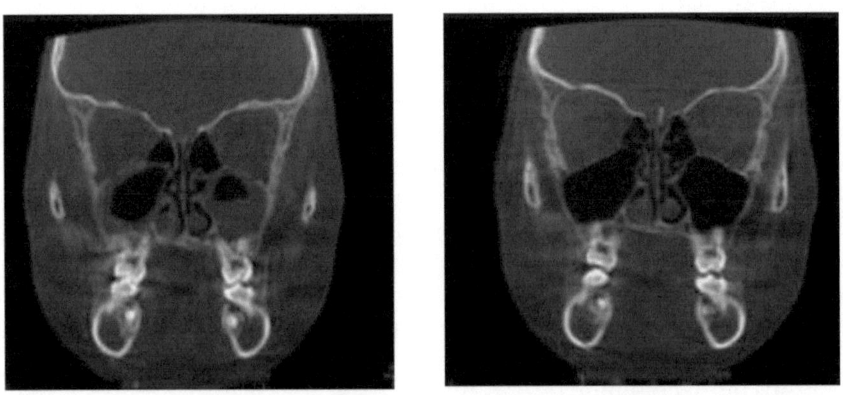

a b

Figure 3.
a: *Case 3: Pre-treatment nasal floor nasal floor width is 15.3 mm;* ***b:*** *Post-treatment width increased to 18.7 m.*

and function through non-surgical remodeling is presumed, there is no clear mechanism of how the sinuses improved during BOAT in these cases. It is possible that the sinusitis resolved through the natural immune response, seasonal changes, through normal craniofacial growth or the placebo effect. However, enlargement of the ostium (>20 mm^2) is thought to decrease sinus NO concentration, as the size of the ostium shows correlation to NO levels [22]. Since the width of the nasal floor increased in these 3 cases (**Figures 1b, 2b** and **3b**), the notion that BOAT involved remodeling of the ostia to within normal limits is yet to be determined.

4. Surgical midfacial expansion

Aside from non-surgical palatal expansion, a plethora of surgical maxillary expansion procedures has become available. One study [23] compared the effects of non-surgical RME with surgically assisted rapid maxillary expansion (SARME). Surprisingly perhaps, there were no differences between the two protocols since nasal cavity width and volume, as well as maxillary width, increased with a concomitant decrease in nasal airway resistance. If non-surgical and surgical techniques yield similar results, one of the questions that currently remains unanswered is, how to minimize or avoid (orthognathic) surgery? To address this subject, Lee et al. [24] described the use of orthodontic screws for mini-screw-assisted rapid maxillary expansion (MARME), since some mistakenly believe that non-surgical palatal expansion relies on unwanted dental tipping rather than actual skeletal expansion. Bearing this in mind, Carlson et al. [25] treated a 19-year-old using MARME. Post-treatment, they reported enlargement in the zygomatic regions and nasal bone regions in association with widening of the circum-maxillary sutures. Indeed, MARME utilizes forces to split the midpalatal suture, which precipitates a midline diastema, an unwanted dental effect. However, insufficient force application may render MARME unsuccessful. Therefore, Suzuki et al. [26] deployed cortical punctures along the midpalatal suture followed by mini-screw insertion to fracture the midpalatal suture by 3-4 mm in an adult patient.

Despite the above variations, the impact of MARME on the upper airway and breathing is not clear. Recently, Abu-Arqub et al. [27] reviewed the effects of MARME on the upper airway in pediatric patients aged 10-17 yrs. They concluded that while short-term improvements were identifiable, no correlation was observed between upper airway morphology and functional parameters, such as nasal airflow and nasal resistance. Similarly, in older patients (mean age 20 yrs.), Yi et al. [28] found that although MARME produced both skeletal and dento-alveolar expansion, there were no changes in the oropharyngeal, palatopharyngeal, and glossopharyngeal regions and the total airway volume remained unaltered on 3D CBCT scans. In another study [29], it was reported that MARME produced an increase in nasal cavity and nasopharyngeal volumes, associated with bony expansion of the nasal floor and maxillary width in young adults (mean age 22.5 yrs.). Thus, when assessing changes on 3D CBCT scans after MARME, the association between skeletal changes and the upper airway remain unclear. Despite these assertions, Singh et al. [30] tested the hypothesis that the upper airway can be improved non-surgically in adults using BOAT. The mean treatment time was 16.5mos. and CBCT scan measurements were taken with no device in the patient's mouth. Their multivariate tests confirmed a significant treatment effect on the upper airway parameters ($p = 0.012$), suggesting that both craniofacial architecture and upper airway morphology can be non-surgically enhanced even in adults. However, this novel approach remains overlooked although further evidence is emerging.

To enhance orthopedics effect induced by MARME, 4 mini-implants with palatal and nasal cortical engagement are sometimes positioned in the palate, when using the maxillary skeletal expander (MSE) technique. Cantarella et al. [31] investigated the effects of this particular protocol on the midpalatal and pterygopalatine sutures in young adults (mean age 17 yrs.). Using CBCT scans, it was found that the midpalatal suture was split slightly asymmetrically, being wider anteriorly than posteriorly. Moreover, pterygopalatine disjunction was revealed in over half of the cases studied, as the pyramidal process of the palatine bone was dislocated from the pterygoid processes. In a similar later study, Cantarella et al. [32] assessed facial changes associated with MSE, again using CBCT scans. Here, it was reported that the zygomatico-maxillary complex showed centrifugal changes with a "center of rotation" located at the fronto-zygomatic suture. Consequently, the inter-zygomatic distances and the fronto-zygomatic angles increased using MSE, but no data on any associated nasopharyngeal airway changes were reported in these particular studies. However, to further locate the center of rotation for the zygomatico-maxillary complex associated with MSE, Cantarella et al. [33] reported that the center of rotation for the zygomatico-maxillary complex could be found more inferiorly, posteriorly and laterally (near the zygomatic process of the temporal bone) compared with their other study [32]. In contrast, Paredes et al. [34] concluded that the center of rotation for the zygomatico-maxillary complex is located at the most infero-lateral point of the zygomatic process of the frontal bone. This variation in the center of rotational displacement could be due to bone deformations that are thought to occur during MSE, which might also explain the occurrence of pterygopalatine dislocation. In fact, Colak et al. [35] evaluated pterygopalatine disarticulation patterns after MSE. The vast majority of cases (> 80%) exhibited pterygopalatine disjunction without direct surgical intervention at this site. The clinical consequences of this iatrogenic fracture, if any, remain undetermined, at least as yet.

Recently, in order to avoid the potential risk of damaging anatomical structures, Cantarella et al. [36] suggested that the deployment of 3D virtual surgical planning using digital data might be advantageous prior to undertaking MSE. Elkenawy et al. [37] were also interested in the biomechanics of MSE. In their study, they noted that over half of approx. 30 adult patients exhibited an asymmetric response following splitting of the midpalatal suture. This result is perhaps not surprising since the midline vomero-maxillary suture would presumably provide an impediment to a symmetric split based *a priori* on fluctuating asymmetry [38]. Indeed, Schwarz et al. [39] examined adult patients for the incidence of nasal septal deviation following SARME. Although no post-operative changes in nasal septal positioning were found, maxillary rotation was associated with an inferior 'rotation' of the palatal vault with a concomitant increase in nasal airway space, although these authors attributed the increases to a decreased thickening of the pre-operative inflamed nasal mucosa. Nonetheless, Abedini et al. [40] were also interested in the soft tissue facial changes induced by MSE. Using 3D stereophotogrammetry, they computed mean 3D soft tissue geometries using techniques similar to those first described by Singh et al. [41, 42] for craniofacial data (**Figure 4**), and were able to demonstrate changes in the paranasal, upper lip, and zygomatic regions of the face associated with MSE. Therefore, clinicians and patients ought to be cognizant of the facial effects associated with MSE prior to embarking upon a treatment plan that putatively targets upper airway inadequacy.

Distraction osteogenesis maxillary expansion (DOME) is another technique that aims to improve the nasal airway changes through widening of the maxilla. Using this approach, Kunkel et al. [43] were able to enlarge the nasal airway volume by 23% on average without pterygomaxillary disjunction being a part of the surgical procedure, which occurs in any case. Despite this drawback, DOME is currently viewed as a reliable procedure to widen the nasal floor in adults with OSA. Using this protocol, the mean apnea-hypopnea index (AHI) was improved, nasal airflow velocity decreased and the mean negative pressures in the nasal, retropalatal, oropharyngeal, and hypopharyngeal airway were reduced, which correlated with a

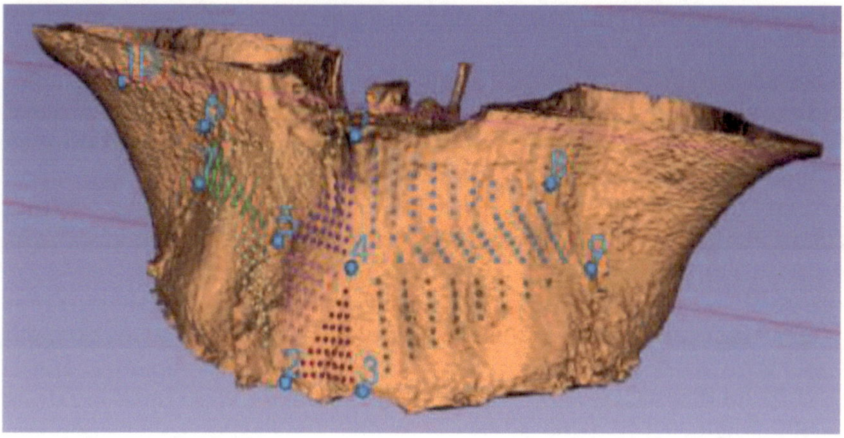

Figure 4.
Using CBCT data, the maxillary complex has been rendered in 3D virtual space and dense correspondence of (colored) landmarks has been computed using the ten homologous landmarks (1–10).

reduction in the AHI, according to Iwasaki et al. [44]. These findings are, however, similar to the well-known results of non-surgical RME using fixed appliance in children. For example, in pediatric cases, Cozza et al. [45] reported that there was a reduction in nasal resistance with increased nasal airflow after RME. Indeed, RME is thought by some to be a comparatively non-invasive, economic treatment option to improve nasal respiration in patients up to at least 30 years of age. Gray [46] considers the medical indications for RME are a deficient nasal airway, septal deformity, recurrent ear infection, and allergic rhinitis, *inter alia*. In a series of over 300 consecutive selected cases, 80% changed their mode of oral breathing to nasal breathing. Thus, the advantages of MSE over RME in terms of nasal airway resistance and anatomical changes in the nasal cavity require further clarification.

5. Nasal airway space, resistance and breathing

In an early study, Warren et al. [47] assessed the effects of non-surgical RME and surgical expansion on nasal airway size. While both procedures improved the nasal airway, approx. 30% of subjects in both groups were unable to eliminate the need for mouth breathing, suggesting that neither RME nor surgical maxillary expansion is justified for nasal breathing purposes alone, likely due to individual variation in response. Bicakci et al. [48] were one of the first to assess the effect of RME on nasal cross-sectional area using acoustic rhinometry, confirming that the overall increase in the cross-sectional area was greater in the RME-treated groups when compared to controls. Around the same time, Ceroni-Compadretti et al. [49] also reported that RME increased both the width of the maxilla and the nasal volume, as measured with acoustic rhinometry. Furthermore, Compadretti et al. [50] deployed rhinomanometry and acoustic rhinometry to assess the function and size of the nasal cavities associated with RME in children. Compared to a control group, the RME treatment group showed an increase in nasal cross-sectional area and volume, as well as a decrease in nasal airway resistance, but the study was unable to confirm the clinical mode of breathing. Likewise, Palaisa et al. [51], using CT scanning, explored the relationship between morphologic changes in nasal area and volume following RME in young patients (8-15 yrs). They reported symmetric increases in both nasal cavity area and volume although the variance in response was again large. Similarly, Oliveira de Felippe et al. [52] concluded that post-expansion, while nasal cross-sectional area increased when measured using acoustic rhinometry, and nasal cavity volume increased using 3D imaging, only 60% of subjects reported subjective improvement in nasal respiration. Therefore, Enoki et al. [53] correctly concluded that RME may lessen nasal resistance but subtle differences in nasal geometry, such as shape changes as opposed to size-changes, may influence success in switching from mouth breathing to nasal respiration.

Currently there is a lack of consensus on the reliability of RME-related procedures in improving nasal functional behaviors, such as changing mouth breathing to nasal breathing predominantly. Hershey et al. [54] noted that patients' subjective opinions on changes in the ability to breathe nasally are not correlated to reductions in treatment-induced nasal resistance, even though RME is effective in reducing nasal resistance to levels consistent with nasal respiration. For example, Doruk et al. [55] found that nearly 60% of 13-yr-olds considered their nasal breathing had improved following RME using subjective evaluation. Earlier, using rhinomanometry, Timms [56] measured nasal airway resistance prior to and after RME in patients aged 10 to 19.5 yrs. On average, a 36% reduction in nasal resistance was reported but this did not correlate with the transpalatal or trans-alar width increases post-expansion. Similarly, Hartgerink et al. [57] surmise that individual variation in nasal resistance values is considerable and that average response variability renders RME unpredictable in terms of decreasing nasal resistance despite evidence of expansion at the anterior nares. In this regard, White et al. [58] reported a mean reduction in nasal airway resistance of approx. 50% after about one-year post-RME. Moreover, they noted that the reduction in nasal airway resistance was correlated to the initial nasal resistance level prior to RME, and that individuals with greater resistance pre-expansion tended to have greater reductions post-treatment. This notion had earlier been investigated using a multidisciplinary approach [59]. Utilizing a combination of RME and oral myofunctional assessment using rhinomanometric measurements, two phenotypes were identified: first, predominantly mouth breathers, showing an average nasal airway resistance decrease of 34%; and second, predominantly nasal breathers with an average nasal airway resistance decrease of <5%. Notably, 75% of predominantly mouth breathers were converted to nasal breathing. Thus, it appears that maxillary deficiency allied with functional deficits needs a tailored approach to be adopted to address the mode of respiration.

It is thought that nasal surgery alone can fail to restore nasal breathing in various cases with maxillary restriction, which is associated with closure of the internal and external nasal valves. In addition, although some now generally agree that RME in both children and adults increases upper airway volume, it remains uncertain whether maxillary expansion improves nasal function. Thus, recently, Iwasaki et al. [60] investigated the efficacy of three RME appliances on nasal ventilation in 10-16 yr. old patients. They reported that RME reduced nasal pressure and nasal airflow velocity, which was accompanied by resolution of nasal obstruction. Nevertheless, Calvo-Henriquez et al. [61] undertook a systematic review on this subject, concluding that there is insufficient evidence to recommend maxillary expansion as a first-line therapy to improve nasal breathing. Despite this assertion, one aspect that remains under-investigated at this juncture is the role of nasal exercises. In the interpretation of numerous studies, it has simply been assumed that an increase or enhancement of anatomical form will result in the desired functional response. But, in their review, Levrini et al. [62] suggest that if RME is combined with functional rehabilitation, the chances of changing a mouth-breathing pattern to nasal respiration are increased. Therefore, the role of respiratory therapists and/or oral myofunctional therapists may need to be extended to include nasal breathing exercises perhaps allied with the use of capnography for biofeedback. In any case, Kiliç and Oktay [63] are of the opinion that while RME increases nasopharyngeal airway dimensions and nasal respiration in pediatric patients exhibiting maxillary constriction and mouth breathing, RME could also be effective on naso-respiratory and sleep-disordered breathing problems in children.

Pirelli et al. [64] evaluated the effect of RME on nasal airway patency and pediatric OSA. On postero-anterior and occlusal radiographic assessment, widening of the midpalatal suture and nasal fossae were confirmed, and restoration of nasal airflow was associated with elimination of obstructive sleep disordered breathing. Therefore, changing the anatomic structure using RME produced significant functional improvement in pediatric patients diagnosed with OSA. On the other hand, Garcez et al. [65] demonstrated the effects of MSE on respiratory function and athletic performance. Using CBCT scans they reported a 6 mm widening of the midpalatal suture and nasomaxillary structures, while the nasal and pharyngeal airways also increased in volume by 30%. In addition, all respiratory indices improved after MSE. Thus, MSE can potentially have a positive influence on both respiratory functions and athletic performance. Recently, Singh et al. [30] also reported a 14% increase in nasal cavity volume achieved non-surgically in adults using a biomimetic oral appliance. Therefore, one of the research question that needs to be addressed now is: Which procedure best suits a particular patient's requirements both safely and effectively? Taking a cohort of cases that have had the same intervention, it should be possible to compute the mean, underlying transformation for a sample of cases. If this transformation can then be applied to a naïve subject, a predictive model can be achieved, assuming the new subject behaves in the same way that the sample did on average. Therefore, the use of mathematical modeling on 3D digital data provides a promising avenue of future research in terms of virtual treatment planning, perhaps incorporating the use of artificial intelligence to inform clinical decision-making.

6. Conclusion

Non-surgical and surgical midfacial expansion techniques are associated with functional sinus changes in the paranasal sinuses as well as changes in nasal airway space, nasal resistance and the mode of breathing. To address the question of which procedure best suits a particular patient's requirements both safely and effectively, the use of mathematical modeling provides a promising approach.

Conflict of interest

Professor G. Dave Singh is Founder and Chief Medical Officer of Vivos Therapeutics, Inc., USA. He is currently collaborating with Stanford University in the development of a craniofacial facility.

Author details

G. Dave Singh
Institute for Craniofacial Sleep Medicine, Highlands Ranch, USA

*Address all correspondence to: drsingh@drdavesingh.com

References

[1] Sereno PC, Martinez RN, Wilson JA, Varricchio DJ, Alcober OA, Larsson HC. Evidence for avian intrathoracic air sacs in a new predatory dinosaur from Argentina. PLoS One. 2008;3:e3303.

[2] Lanteri V, Farronato M, Ugolini A, Cossellu G, Gaffuri F, Parisi FMR, Cavagnetto D, Abate A, Maspero C. Volumetric changes in the upper airways after rapid and slow maxillary expansion in growing patients: A case-control study. Materials (Basel). 2020;13:2239.

[3] Garrett BJ, Caruso JM, Rungcharassaeng K, Farrage JR, Kim JS, Taylor GD. Skeletal effects to the maxilla after rapid maxillary expansion assessed with cone-beam computed tomography. Am J Orthod Dentofacial Orthop. 2008;134:8-9.

[4] Pangrazio-Kulbersh V, Wine P, Haughey M, Pajtas B, Kaczynski R. Cone beam computed tomography evaluation of changes in the naso-maxillary complex associated with two types of maxillary expanders. Angle Orthod. 2012;82:448-457.

[5] Almuzian M, Ju X, Almukhtar A, Ayoub A, Al-Muzian L, McDonald JP. Does rapid maxillary expansion affect nasopharyngeal airway? A prospective Cone Beam Computerised Tomography (CBCT) based study. Surgeon. 2018;16: 1-11.

[6] Pamporakis P, Nevzatoğlu Ş, Küçükkeleş N. Three-dimensional alterations in pharyngeal airway and maxillary sinus volumes in Class III maxillary deficiency subjects undergoing orthopedic facemask treatment. Angle Orthod. 2014;84:701-707.

[7] Onem-Ozbilen E, Yilmaz HN, Kucukkeles N. Comparison of the effects of rapid maxillary expansion and alternate rapid maxillary expansion and constriction protocols followed by facemask therapy. Korean J Orthod. 2019;49:49-58.

[8] Erdur EA, Yıldırım M, Karatas RMC, Akin M. Effects of symmetric and asymmetric rapid maxillary expansion treatments on pharyngeal airway and sinus volume. Angle Orthod. 2020;90: 425-431.

[9] Machado-Júnior AJ, Crespo AN. Expansion of the maxilla in adults with OSAS: myth or reality? Sleep Med. 2020;65:170-171.

[10] Kavand G, Lagravère M, Kula K, Stewart K, Ghoneima A. Retrospective CBCT analysis of airway volume changes after bone-borne vs tooth-borne rapid maxillary expansion. Angle Orthod. 2019;89:566-574.

[11] Singh GD, Kim HN. Changes in pneumatization of the maxillary air sinuses in Korean adults following biomimetic oral appliance therapy. World J Otorhinolaryngol Head Neck Surg. 2020 doi.org/10.1016/j.wjorl.2020.07.007.

[12] Maniscalco M, Bianco A, Mazzarella G, Motta A. Recent Advances on Nitric Oxide in the Upper Airways. Curr Med Chem. 2016;23:2736-2745.

[13] Jankowski R, Nguyen DT, Poussel M, Chenuel B, Gallet P, Rumeau C. Sinusology. Eur Ann Otorhinolaryngol Head Neck Dis. 2016;133:263-268.

[14] Lundberg JO, Weitzberg E, Rinder J, Rudehill A, Jansson O, Wiklund NP, Lundberg JM, Alving K. Calcium-independent and steroid-resistant nitric oxide synthase activity in human paranasal sinus mucosa. Eur Respir J. 1996;9:1344-1347.

[15] Andersson JA, Cervin A, Lindberg S, Uddman R, Cardell LO. The paranasal sinuses as reservoirs for nitric oxide. Acta Otolaryngol. 2002;122: 861-865.

[16] Runer T, Cervin A, Lindberg S, Uddman R. Nitric oxide is a regulator of mucociliary activity in the upper respiratory tract. Otolaryngol Head Neck Surg. 1998;119:278-287.

[17] Deja M, Busch T, Bachmann S, Riskowski K, Campean V, Wiedmann B, Schwabe M, Hell B, Pfeilschifter J, Falke KJ, Lewandowski K. Reduced nitric oxide in sinus epithelium of patients with radiologic maxillary sinusitis and sepsis. Am J Respir Crit Care Med. 2003;168:281-286.

[18] Naraghi M, Deroee AF, Ebrahimkhani M, Kiani S, Dehpour A. Nitric oxide: a new concept in chronic sinusitis pathogenesis. Am J Otolaryngol. 2007;28:334-337.

[19] Degano B, Génestal M, Serrano E, Rami J, Arnal JF. Effect of treatment on maxillary sinus and nasal nitric oxide concentrations in patients with nosocomial maxillary sinusitis. Chest 2005;128:1699-1705.

[20] Wen YS, Lin CY, Yang KD, Hung CH, Chang YJ, Tsai YG. Nasal nitric oxide is a useful biomarker for acute unilateral maxillary sinusitis in pediatric allergic rhinitis: A prospective observational cohort study. World Allergy Organ J. 2019;12:100027.

[21] Hwang H, Hwang C, West J, Singh GD. Changes in pediatric paranasal sinuses following biomimetic oral appliance therapy: 3 case reports. Cranio. 2019:1-6.

[22] Kirihene RK, Rees G, Wormald PJ. The influence of the size of the maxillary sinus ostium on the nasal and sinus nitric oxide levels. Am J Rhinol. 2002;16:261-264.

[23] Basciftci FA, Mutlu N, Karaman AI, Malkoc S, Küçükkolbasi H. Does the timing and method of rapid maxillary expansion have an effect on the changes in nasal dimensions? Angle Orthod. 2002;72:118-123.

[24] Lee KJ, Park YC, Park JY, Hwang WS. Miniscrew-assisted nonsurgical palatal expansion before orthognathic surgery for a patient with severe mandibular prognathism. Am J Orthod Dentofacial Orthop. 2010;137: 830-839.

[25] Carlson C, Sung J, McComb RW, Machado AW, Moon W. Microimplant-assisted rapid palatal expansion appliance to orthopedically correct transverse maxillary deficiency in an adult. Am J Orthod Dentofacial Orthop. 2016;149:716-728.

[26] Suzuki SS, Braga LFS, Fujii DN, Moon W, Suzuki H. Corticopuncture Facilitated Microimplant-Assisted Rapid Palatal Expansion. Case Rep Dent. 2018;1392895.

[27] Abu-Arqub S, Mehta S, Iverson MG, Yadav S, Upadhyay M, Almuzian M. Does Mini Screw Assisted Rapid Palatal Expansion (MARPE) have an influence on airway and breathing in middle-aged children and adolescents? A systematic review. Int Orthod. 2021;19:37-50.

[28] Yi F, Liu S, Lei L, Liu O, Zhang L, Peng Q, Lu Y. Changes of the upper airway and bone in microimplant-assisted rapid palatal expansion: A cone-beam computed tomography (CBCT) study. J Xray Sci Technol. 2020;28:271-283.

[29] Li Q, Tang H, Liu X, Luo Q, Jiang Z, Martin D, Guo J. Comparison of dimensions and volume of upper airway before and after mini-implant assisted rapid maxillary expansion. Angle Orthod. 2020;90:432-441.

[30] Singh GD, Kim HN, Kim SH, Wang L. 3D craniofacial and upper

airway changes after biomimetic oral appliance therapy in Korean adults. Otorhinolaryngol Head Neck Surg. 2021;6:1-7.

[31] Cantarella D, Dominguez-Mompell R, Mallya SM, Moschik C, Pan HC, Miller J, Moon W. Changes in the midpalatal and pterygopalatine sutures induced by micro-implant-supported skeletal expander, analyzed with a novel 3D method based on CBCT imaging. Prog Orthod. 2017;18:34.

[32] Cantarella D, Dominguez-Mompell R, Moschik C, Mallya SM, Pan HC, Alkahtani MR, Elkenawy I, Moon W. Midfacial changes in the coronal plane induced by microimplant-supported skeletal expander, studied with cone-beam computed tomography images. Am J Orthod Dentofacial Orthop. 2018;154:337-345.

[33] Cantarella D, Dominguez-Mompell R, Moschik C, Sfogliano L, Elkenawy I, Pan HC, Mallya SM, Moon W. Zygomaticomaxillary modifications in the horizontal plane induced by micro-implant-supported skeletal expander, analyzed with CBCT images. Prog Orthod. 2018;19:41.

[34] Paredes, N., Colak, O., Sfogliano, L. et al. Differential assessment of skeletal, alveolar, and dental components induced by microimplant-supported midfacial skeletal expander (MSE), utilizing novel angular measurements from the fulcrum. Prog Orthod. 2020;21:18.

[35] Colak O, Paredes NA, Elkenawy I, Torres M, Bui J, Jahangiri S, Moon W. Tomographic assessment of palatal suture opening pattern and pterygopalatine suture disarticulation in the axial plane after midfacial skeletal expansion. Prog Orthod. 2020;21:21.

[36] Cantarella D, Savio G, Grigolato L, Zanata P, Berveglieri C, Lo Giudice A, Isola G, Del Fabbro M, Moon W. A New Methodology for the Digital Planning of Micro-Implant-Supported Maxillary Skeletal Expansion. Med Devices (Auckl). 2020;13:93-106.

[37] Elkenawy I, Fijany L, Colak O, Paredes NA, Gargoum A, Abedini S, Cantarella D, Dominguez-Mompell R, Sfogliano L, Moon W. An assessment of the magnitude, parallelism, and asymmetry of micro-implant-assisted rapid maxillary expansion in non-growing patients. Prog Orthod. 2020;21:42.

[38] Auffray, J.C.; Debat, V.; Alibert, P. Shape asymmetry and developmental stability. In: Chaplain MAJ, Singh GD, McLachlan JC, editors. On Growth and Form: Spatio-Temporal Pattern Formation in Biology. Chichester: Wiley; 1999. p. 309-324.

[39] Schwarz GM, Thrash WJ, Byrd DL, Jacobs JD. Tomographic assessment of nasal septal changes following surgical-orthodontic rapid maxillary expansion. Am J Orthod. 1985;87:39-45. doi: 10.1016/0002-9416(85)90172-1.

[40] Abedini S, Elkenawy I, Kim E, Moon W. Three-dimensional soft tissue analysis of the face following micro-implant-supported maxillary skeletal expansion. Prog Orthod. 2018;19:46.

[41] Singh GD, McNamara JA Jr., Lozanoff S. Morphometry of the cranial base in subjects with Class III malocclusion. J. Dent. Res. 1997;76: 694-703.

[42] Singh GD, Levy-Bercowski D, Yañez MA, Santiago PE. Three-dimensional facial morphology following surgical repair of unilateral cleft lip and palate in patients after nasoalveolar molding. Orthod Craniofac Res. 2007;10: 161-166.

[43] Kunkel M, Ekert O, Wagner W. [Changes in the nasal airway by transverse distraction of the maxilla].

Mund Kiefer Gesichtschir. 1999;3:12-6. [Article in German]

[44] Iwasaki T, Yoon A, Guilleminault C, Yamasaki Y, Liu SY. How does distraction osteogenesis maxillary expansion (DOME) reduce severity of obstructive sleep apnea? Sleep Breath. 2020;24:287-296.

[45] Cozza P, Di Girolamo S, Ballanti F, Panfilio F. Orthodontist-otorhinolaryngologist: an inter disciplinary approach to solve otitis media. Eur J Paediatr Dent. 2007;8: 83-88.

[46] Gray LP. Results of 310 cases of rapid maxillary expansion selected for medical reasons. J Laryngol Otol. 1975;89:601-614.

[47] Warren DW, Hershey HG, Turvey TA, Hinton VA, Hairfield WM. The nasal airway following maxillary expansion. Am J Orthod Dentofacial Orthop. 1987;91:111-116.

[48] Bicakci AA, Agar U, Sökücü O, Babacan H, Doruk C. Nasal airway changes due to rapid maxillary expansion timing. Angle Orthod. 2005;75:1-6.

[49] Ceroni Compadretti G, Tasca I, Alessandri-Bonetti G, Peri S, D'Addario A. Acoustic rhinometric measurements in children undergoing rapid maxillary expansion. Int J Pediatr Otorhinolaryngol. 2006;70:27-34.

[50] Compadretti GC, Tasca I, Bonetti GA. Nasal airway measurements in children treated by rapid maxillary expansion. Am J Rhinol. 2006;20: 385-393.

[51] Palaisa J, Ngan P, Martin C, Razmus T. Use of conventional tomography to evaluate changes in the nasal cavity with rapid palatal expansion. Am J Orthod Dentofacial Orthop. 2007;132:458-466.

[52] Oliveira De Felippe NL, Da Silveira AC, Viana G, Kusnoto B, Smith B, Evans CA. Relationship between rapid maxillary expansion and nasal cavity size and airway resistance: short- and long-term effects. Am J Orthod Dentofacial Orthop. 2008;134: 370-382.

[53] Enoki C, Valera FC, Lessa FC, Elias AM, Matsumoto MA, Anselmo-Lima WT. Effect of rapid maxillary expansion on the dimension of the nasal cavity and on nasal air resistance. Int J Pediatr Otorhino laryngol. 2006;70:1225-1230.

[54] Hershey HG, Stewart BL, Warren DW. Changes in nasal airway resistance associated with rapid maxillary expansion. Am J Orthod. 1976;69:274-284.

[55] Doruk C, Sökücü O, Sezer H, Canbay EI. Evaluation of nasal airway resistance during rapid maxillary expansion using acoustic rhinometry. Eur J Orthod. 2004;26:397-401.

[56] Timms DJ. The effect of rapid maxillary expansion on nasal airway resistance. Br J Orthod. 1986; 13:221-228.

[57] Hartgerink DV, Vig PS, Abbott DW. The effect of rapid maxillary expansion on nasal airway resistance. Am J Orthod Dentofacial Orthop. 1987;92:381-389.

[58] White BC, Woodside DG, Cole P. The effect of rapid maxillary expansion on nasal airway resistance. J Otolaryngol. 1989;18(4):137-143.

[59] Wollens AG, Goffart Y, Lismonde P, Limme M. [Therapeutic maxillary expansion]. Rev Belge Med Dent (1984) 1991;46:51-8. [Article in French]

[60] Iwasaki T, Papageorgiou SN, Yamasaki Y, Ali Darendeliler M, Papadopoulou AK. Nasal ventilation and rapid maxillary expansion (RME):

a randomized trial. Eur J Orthod. 2021 Feb 10:cjab001.

[61] Calvo-Henriquez C, Megias-Barrera J, Chiesa-Estomba C, Lechien JR, Maldonado Alvarado B, Ibrahim B, Suarez-Quintanilla D, Kahn S, Capasso R. The impact of maxillary expansion on adults' nasal breathing: A systematic review and meta-analysis. Am J Rhinol Allergy. 2021:1945892421995350. doi: 10.1177/1945892421995350. Epub ahead of print.

[62] Levrini L, Lorusso P, Caprioglio A, Magnani A, Diaféria G, Bittencourt L, Bommarito S. Model of oronasal rehabilitation in children with obstructive sleep apnea syndrome undergoing rapid maxillary expansion: Research review. Sleep Sci. 2014;7: 225-233.

[63] Kiliç N, Oktay H. Effects of rapid maxillary expansion on nasal breathing and some naso-respiratory and breathing problems in growing children: a literature review. Int J Pediatr Otorhinolaryngol. 2008;72:1595-1601.

[64] Pirelli P, Saponara M, Attanasio G. Obstructive Sleep Apnoea Syndrome (OSAS) and rhino-tubaric disfunction in children: therapeutic effects of RME therapy. Prog Orthod. 2005;6:48-61.

[65] Garcez AS, Suzuki SS, Storto CJ, Cusmanich KG, Elkenawy I, Moon W. Effects of maxillary skeletal expansion on respiratory function and sport performance in a para-athlete – A case report. Phys Ther Sport 2019;36:70-77.

Chapter 6

Maxillary Sinus in Dental Implantology

Nikolay Uzunov and Elena Bozhikova

Abstract

Dental implants have significantly increased prosthetic options for the edentulous patient. Implant placement in the posterior maxilla may often be hampered due to anatomical limitations, inadequate height and width, and poor bone quality. After tooth extraction, three-dimensional physiological resorption and sinus expansion take place and reduce the volume of the alveolar ridge. The concomitant actions of alveolar atrophy and sinus pneumatization reconstruct the subantral alveolar segment into a low, shallow, and sloped ridge which is incapable to accommodate dental implants and bear the functional strains. Advanced maxillary resorption can be managed by several surgical options, the most popular of which is maxillary sinus floor elevation. The chapter discusses recent advancements in bone biology and biomechanics in the light of alveolar atrophy and the impact of anatomy on maxillary sinus floor elevation as a treatment modality for the partially or totally edentulous patient.

Keywords: maxillary sinus floor elevation, dental implants, maxillary atrophy, maxillary pneumatization, maxillary edentulism

1. Introduction

Dental implants (DI) have significantly increased prosthetic options for the edentulous patient. However, implant placement in the posterior maxilla is often hampered by anatomical limitations such as inadequate vertical and buccopalatal dimensions, poor bone quality, thin or missing cortex, and undercuts. Following tooth extraction, three-dimensional resorption of the alveolar ridge takes place and reduces its' dimensions; in addition, the periosteum of the maxillary sinus (MS) can exhibit an increase in osteoclastic activity. The latter can aggravate the physiological process of maxillary sinus pneumatization (MSP) or aeration. The concomitant actions of postextraction alveolar atrophy (AA) and MSP worsen the subantral alveolar dimensions in short terms and makes doubtful the prosthetic rehabilitation with DIs, as adequate bone height and width are mandatory to implant treatment [1–4]. The principal solution for alveolar insufficiency is to augment the distal maxilla. Several surgical approaches have the potential to improve the subantral osseous environment to prepare the edentulous segment for the accommodation of DI, and the most popular is maxillary sinus floor elevation (MSFE).

2. Alveolar atrophy after tooth extraction

Alveolar atrophy is defined as loss or diminution of supportive alveolar bone due to loss of teeth or to function, trauma, reduced blood supply, or unknown cause [5]. The most common reason for AA is the alveolar resorption after tooth loss [6]. Removal of a tooth is followed by remodeling and reduction of the buccolingual and apicocoronal dimensions of the edentulous segment and results in a shorter and narrower alveolar ridge [6–10]. Unaddressed, postextraction AA develops through the whole lifespan of the person (**Figure 1**). Jaws with progressive bone loss are subjected to continuing anatomical make-over that alters normal orofacial tissue configuration which may affect the social integration and realization of the affected individuals. In advanced AA cases, adequate anatomical, functional, and esthetic rehabilitation is highly complicated.

2.1 Physiology and biomechanics of bone atrophy

In 1881 Wilhelm Roux suggested that the natural forces acting on the alveolar ridge are reduced after tooth loss. As result, less bone is needed to maintain function, and, consequently, the body gets rid of the non-functioning structures. It was concluded that loss of alveolar bone after tooth removal is an example of disuse atrophy. Eleven years later Wolff's law stated that bone tissue adapts its mass and architecture to the mechanical demands [10].

It was understood that loads play a key role in bone biology. The principles of biomechanics were applied to present bone mass maintenance and resorption as a reaction to continuously repeated loading impetus. The daily stress stimulus theory of bone adaptation was formulated to describe the loading conditions necessary to support bone mass and recognized the stress/strain magnitude and loading cycle number as sufficient to define an appropriate maintenance loading signal [11]. Frost [12] published a hypothesis on a provisional general model of the skeleton's mechanostat. According to this hypothesis, the mechanostat spans the biological distance

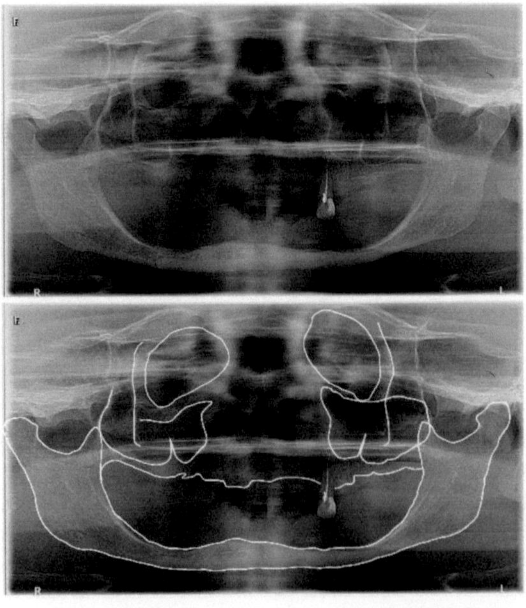

Figure 1.
Advanced maxillary and mandibular alveolar atrophy in a 64-year-old male.

between organs and macromolecules and can be applied to "all organs and tissues, including bone, made wholly or in part from the basic tissues". It was proposed that "interlocking negative feedback loops" provide mechanical-usage-dedicated message traffic routes on which nonmechanical agents could act to optimize postnatal skeletal adaptations to varied mechanical and nonmechanical challenges, and treatments of disease [12]. The understanding that mechanical stimuli can be transferred to the bone by a signaling network was further developed by Burger and Klein-Nulend in the mechanotransduction concept. They pointed that the osteocytes function as mechanosensory cells of osseous tissues and explained the capacity of bone to change its mass and structure in response to mechanical demands within specific cellular mechanisms [13].

For a long time, the contribution of osteocytes to bone biology was undervalued as they were accepted as terminal stage cells of the osteoblastic lineage. Recent investigations addressed the osteocytes and their role in bone orchestration and revealed that they may have mechanosensory, endocrine, and homeostatic activity.

Osteocytes are the most abundant bone cells and the only cells embedded in the bone mineral matrix. After being entrapped in bone, the osteocytes are housed within lacunae and connect to each other by cytoplasmic processes hosted in channels called canaliculi. The lacunae and the canaliculi form a three-dimensional (3D) network named the lacuno-canalicular network (LCN). In the light of mechanotransduction, the strains in bone accumulated under loads may induce a strain-derived flow of interstitial fluid through the LCN which mechanically activates the osteocytes to respond to the loading stimuli and ensure the transport of cell signaling molecules, nutrients, and waste products. This explains local bone gain, loss, and remodeling, in response to fatigue damage, as cellular and intercellular activity supervised by the mechanosensitive osteocytes [13]. The LCN is a negative imprint of the cellular network in the bone and its morphology is considered to play a central role in bone mechanosensation and mechanotransduction [14]. Within the LCN, the osteocytes can transport nutrients, biochemical signals, and hormonal stimuli, enabling the integration of the information between and interaction with other bone cells [15].

The general existence and micro-anatomy of the LCN have been known for a long time. The connections of the osteocyte network with other regions of the body [16] and its importance for phosphate metabolism [13, 15] were debated in recent research [17, 18]. As endocrine cells, osteocytes have an impact on many organs [16]. They communicate with the kidney through the factor FGF23 [19], and with the brain, through the expression of leptin [20]. The osteocytes could be regulators of bone resorption by secreting the Receptor activator of NF-κB ligand (RANKL) [21] and control bone formation by producing WNT1 glycoprotein [22, 23]. They contribute to fat metabolism by secreting sclerostin, which promotes the increase of beige adipogenesis [22], and influence hematopoiesis by the adjustment of the endosteal microenvironment through the release of soluble factors [24].

The connectivity between osteocytes themselves is of crucial importance to understand bone health [17]. Within the complex communication between cells, the osteocyte network acts as a mechano-sensory organ [25]. Through sensing the fluid flow in LCN and sclerostin expression, the osteocytes regulate bone's mechanobiological adaptation and remodeling [26]. The hypothesis of the LCN connectome, paralleling the neurosensory connectome, is emerging from the complex LCN organization and wealth of connections within the bone and with other organs [17].

It is important to distinguish between the LCN and the osteocyte network as a connected cell network. However, most of the functions of the osteocyte network can only be understood in the interplay between the "biological" cell network and the "material" porosity in the mineralized matrix [25]. In human osteons, canaliculi that are not oriented towards the Haversian canal were found to be co-aligned with the preferred matrix orientation. The pericanalicular matrix in the immediate vicinity of the cell processes was shown to be disordered and more mineralized with increased thickness of the mineral particles incorporated in the collagen matrix. This higher mineral content around the canaliculi is remarkable in the context of the osteocytes' contribution to calcium and phosphate metabolism. Recent evidence revived the almost forgotten idea of osteocytic osteolysis. Due to the high surface area of the LCN and the small distance from the LCN to any point in the bone matrix, osteocytes have easy access to the bone mineral and can demineralize bone. The role of osteocytes as mechanosensors and orchestrators of bone remodeling depends crucially on the interaction between cell network and porous network.

The fluid flow hypothesis assumes that mechanical loads squeeze interstitial bone fluid through the pericellular space between the cell processes and bodies in the canaliculi and lacunae. The osteocytes and their processes sense the shear forces caused by the fluid flow, and it seems that the cell processes are more mechanosensitive than the cell body. The details of the fluid flow and the resulting shear forces do not only depend on the connectivity and the irregular shape of the canaliculi, but also on how the cells deform due to the flow and how the cell processes are anchored on the canaliculi walls [17]. More recently, a newly discovered cell type, osteomorphs, was proved to participate in bone resorption and remodeling. It was shown that osteoclasts recycle via osteomorphs and that the latter may be targeted for the treatment of resorptive skeletal diseases [27].

2.2 Biomechanics of alveolar bone

It was confirmed that the grounds of understanding bone physiology are the osteocyte reactions to stress stimuli, inducing bone resorption, remodeling, and adaptation, on one hand, and biomechanics, on the other. Several investigations addressed the biomechanics of bone adaptation. Qin et al. examined a turkey ulna model of disuse osteopenia to determine whether the daily stress theory of bone adaptation can be applied to conditions of very high numbers of loading cycles at very low strain magnitudes [28]. They found that the strain stimulus needed per day to maintain bone mass could be expressed by the formula

$$y = 10^{2.28}\left(5.6 - \log_{10} x\right)^{1.5} \qquad (1)$$

where x is the number of loading cycles per day and y is the strain magnitude. The results proved the strong antiresorptive influence of mechanical loading identifying a threshold for a daily loading cycle regimen near 70 microstrain of approximately 100,000 strain cycles, and suggest that the strain frequency or strain rate associated with the loading stimulus must also play a critical role in the mechanism by which bone, as a tissue, responds to mechanical loads.

In 2012 Hansson and Halldin tested such experiments and investigated, in the light of mechanics of materials, the correlation between established principles of bone physiology and the changes in the dimensions of the alveolar ridge after tooth extraction [10]. Their considerations were based on the mathematical presentation of principal stresses and strains acting on the mandible as a beam subjected to loads and, also, the differences in the response of cancellous and cortical bone to strains. Data analysis from clinical and experimental investigations on the effects of strains on lamellar organization and orientation of cancellous bone [29–31], the alignment of the Haversian systems in cortical bones [32], and bone mass dependence on the magnitude of strains, was integrated with experimental findings on the healing of postextraction sockets and resorption of the empty alveolar ridge. One month after tooth extraction the empty socket is filled with woven bone. Three months later the woven bone is substituted by a cortical ridge-like structure consisting of lamellar and woven bone which, in turn, is substituted in the sixth month by an alveolar ridge constructed of lamellar bone and bone marrow [33]. It was also pointed that the resorption of the buccal and lingual alveolar walls occurs in two overlapping phases; in the first phase, the bundle bone is resorbed and replaced with woven bone, while the second phase includes resorption from the outer surface of both bone walls, and that the resorption is larger at the buccal aspect of the ridge than at the lingual aspect [34–37].

Considering the mandible as a beam subjected to strains, i.e., bending moments, the authors speculated that the extraction socket will gradually be filled with lamellar and cancellous bone, which will make the healed extraction site stiffer both to horizontal and vertical bending. The bending moments remain unchanged and, consecutively, the bone strains will be reduced [10]. Reduced bone strains result in bone loss [28, 38]. Speculation on bone physiology and biomechanics brings the conclusion that alveolar and jaw resorption is a natural result of the fundamental physiological principle of adaptation of bone mass and bone structure to the levels and frequencies of strain [10].

3. Practical aspects of alveolar atrophy of the distal maxilla

3.1 Alveolar atrophy and dental implants

Masticatory forces are distributed to the skull through the fronto-maxillary (frontonasal), the zygomatico-maxillary, and the pterygomaxillary pillars, and the palatine arch [38, 39]. DI placement requires bony structures with adequate volume, and [1] therefore, the volume of the alveolar crest is a principal consideration for DI treatment. In the distal maxilla, the subantral height, i.e., the height of the inferior MS wall, and width of the alveolar span are of crucial importance in treatment planning.

After tooth loss, the alveolar bone undergoes fast remodeling that leads to horizontal and vertical decrease of crestal dimensions [6, 40]. When, after tooth extraction, the alveolus is occupied by bone, or by DI and bone, the stiffness of the edentulous span will be increased. With unchanged loads, increased stiffness implies reduced strains, and the strain stimulus needed to maintain bone mass is no longer reached. The biological response to this is to remove bone and reduce the bony volume. Therefore, placing a DI in the empty alveolus will increase alveolar stiffness, and, theoretically, immediate DI placement into fresh extraction sockets should not be expected to prevent the dimensional reduction of the alveolar ridge [10].

Clinical trials and systematic reviews demonstrated that horizontal and vertical resorption is more pronounced at the buccal aspect of the ridge than at the lingual aspect [34, 35, 37, 41–43] and that the horizontal reduction is greater than the loss in height [34]. The consequence of a greater vertical bone loss buccally than lingually is a ridge that is sloped in the lingual to the buccal direction (**Figure 2**). A new "tug-of-war" hypothesis explains the more pronounced buccal resorption with the forces acting at the empty socket after tooth loss and the activity of the myofibroblasts as their pull is directed from the buccal and palatal edges towards the center of the alveolus. Since the balance depends on the relative mass of the two edges, the thin buccal wall would be the one to cede under the tension of the granulation tissue [44].

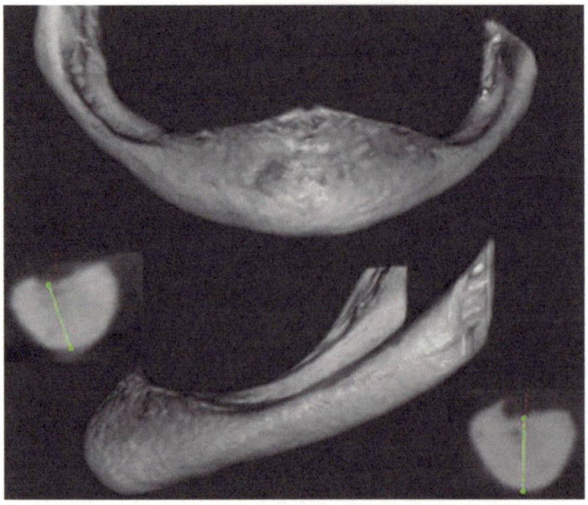

Figure 2.
Advanced alveolar atrophy of the mandible resulting in a sloped alveolar ridge.

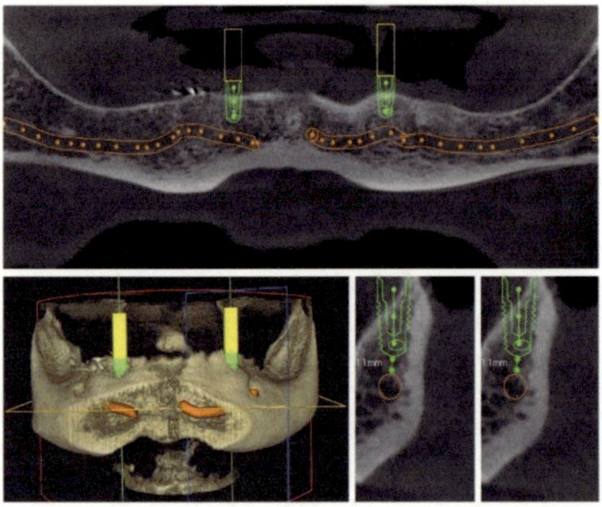

Figure 3.
The sloped alveolar ridge does not allow for placement of DI without ridge augmentation.

In cases with a sloped alveolar ridge, the insertion of standard DI might not be optimal (**Figure 3**). Implant placement in level with the lingual bone margin may result in compromised esthetics. If DI instead is placed at a level with the buccal margin, the lingual marginal bone is at risk to be resorbed due to insufficient strain stimulus. In a clinical study, DI with a sloped marginal contour was used in cases with an alveolar crest sloped in lingual to buccal direction. Both the mean buccal marginal bone level change and the mean lingual marginal bone level change after 16 weeks amounted to −0.2 mm. Thus, the installation of a DI with a sloped marginal contour may be a treatment option in cases where the alveolar ridge is sloped in lingual to the buccal direction [10, 45].

3.2 Atrophy of the distal maxilla

The above line of arguments can be applied to the maxilla with its complicated anatomy, lesser bone density, and aeration. Disuse atrophy creates a sloped and reduced in height alveolar profile, constructed mostly from soft trabecular bone. Moreover, the edentulous maxillary posterior sextants were shown to have the least amount of residual bone height compared with other edentulous regions of the maxilla and, therefore, represent one of the most critical areas to be rehabilitated by an implant-supported prosthesis [46]. In addition, the postextraction bone resorption in the distal maxilla may be associated with MSP, which may contribute to a further decrease of the available bone volume for DI placement [47].

3.3 Residual alveolar height of the distal maxilla and maxillary sinus pneumatization

The aeration of the paranasal cavities is a physiological process the effect of which is an increase in sinus volume and decrease in the volume of the surrounding bone during growth. MSP adds additional three-dimensional reduction to the postextraction alveolar resorption in the distal maxilla (**Figure 4**) [2, 40].

The MS begins its development in the 10th week. At the time of birth, the sinus is already pneumatized and increases in size through continuous MSP during the whole life of the individual [48, 49]. With the eruption of the permanent dentition, MSP is paused, and the sinus reaches 4–5 mm below the nasal cavity as an alveolar recess [50]. The variations in MS volume and dimensions among individuals and tooth position are significant. The alveolar recess can project between adjacent teeth or between the roots of the same tooth [51]. This is often observed between the roots of the first and the second molar which have a very close relationship to the sinus floor [52–55]. Tooth loss unlocks sinus aeration again and its effect is added to the effect of the postextraction alveolar resorption.

Several studies reported significant MSP after tooth extraction and accepted that alveolar bone height in the edentulous distal maxilla is a result of the concomitant actions of crestal atrophy and apical sinus enlargement. The anatomical and pathological peculiarities of the distal maxilla contribute to the MS expansion after removal of the first and the second upper molars. The ultimate anatomical

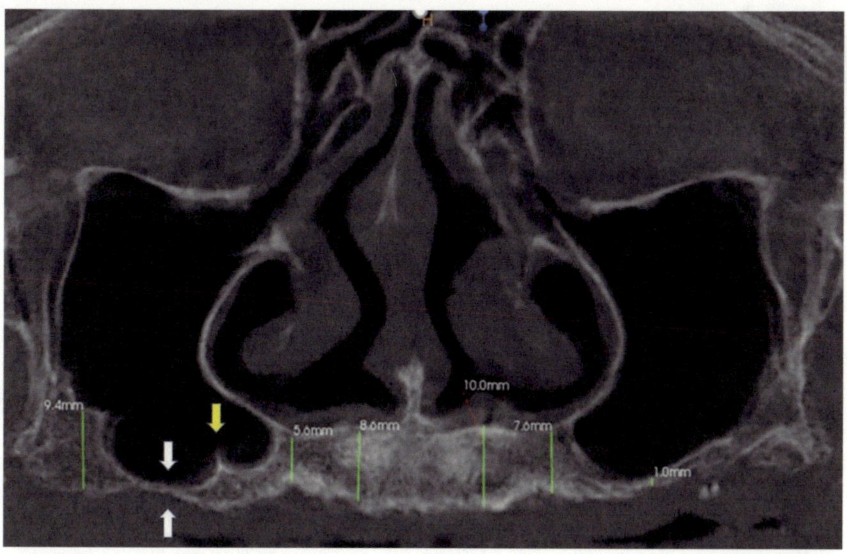

Figure 4.
Advanced alveolar atrophy and pneumatization of the distal maxilla. Note that the subantral height is 1 mm on the left and even less on the right (white arrows). The sinus pneumatization extends into the premolar region and lies beneath the nasal floor bilaterally approximating the canines. A well-defined sinus floor septum is found in the right (yellow arrow). The sinus drainage is doubtful on both sides, due to thickened mucosa.

consideration is the proximity between the root apices of these teeth and the sinus floor [2, 40, 55–57]. This means that the height of the bony roofs of the alveoli of the upper molars, i.e., the thickness of the inferior sinus wall, is anatomically small, and, in turn, can be more readily reduced by AA and MSP even in cases without preceding pathology in or trauma to this region. The same is the cause for asymptomatic cortical bone fractures of the alveolar roof during upper molar extraction. Extensive ridge atrophy and MSP can be provoked by the removal of teeth which roots elevate the sinus floor or are enveloped by a superiorly curving floor. Multiple extractions within the same segment initiate more aggressive AA and MSP and reduce considerably ridge volume and resistance to the loading stimuli. Considering that the causes for tooth loss are mainly periapical and/or periodontal pathology, and trauma, it becomes clearer why postextraction alveolar resorption is often accelerated at the distal maxilla and why the loss of maxillary molars is considered to provoke excessive MSP [2, 40, 57–60]. It is not still completely understood how much atrophy and MSP contribute actually to the total loss of bony height [2, 61, 62].

Other studies could not confirm MS expansion after tooth loss [63, 64]. The role of residual ridge resorption and MSP was recently addressed in the overall maxillary bony atrophy using principal components analysis [65]. They found that most of the bone loss occurring in the alveolar process is caused by disuse atrophy due to edentulism and concluded that while the alveolar crest is changed by tooth loss, the MS is not, which refers sinus depth to anatomical variation independent of dentition. Prolonged edentulism in the maxillary molar region leads to centripetal and, to minor degrees, to centrifugal ridge resorption. Minor MSP occurs in the walls thinning the buccal and palatal aspects, which may be attributed to the absence of roots or variation in force transmission to the zygomatic or the nasopalatal buttresses [65].

The reasons for MSP after tooth extraction are still debated. With tooth loss, the functional forces which are normally transferred to the bone are weakened which can cause a shift in the physiologic bone remodeling to a resorptive pattern [58]. Previous studies demonstrated a downward expansion of the MS after tooth loss and showed that it was larger if the extracted tooth was surrounded by a superiorly curved sinus floor [2, 66–68].

In conclusion, advanced alveolar resorption constitutes a sloped alveolar ridge with inadequate bone volume and quality that limits conventional DI treatment. The bone density in the distal maxilla is the lowest in comparison to other jaw regions. The edentulous upper molar alveolar ridge presents with a thin cortex and a loose trabecular subcortical bone. This means that the biomechanical properties and the healing potential of this segment may be insufficient to secure primary DI stability and graft consolidation.

4. Maxillary sinus floor elevation

Treatment limitations present functional and esthetic impairments to the affected individuals. In such cases, the rehabilitation of the altered jaw segments necessitates the reconstruction of the missing dentoalveolar tissues. An increasing number of patients with edentulous posterior maxilla needs bone and soft tissue augmentation procedures to allow proper DI placement and achieve satisfactory results [46].

Maxillary sinus floor elevation (MSFE) is a treatment concept the purpose of which is volume augmentation of the distal maxilla to enhance the prosthetic rehabilitation of partial or total maxillary edentulism with DI. The goal is achieved with two basic surgical techniques and their variations that share a common key point which is to intrude the subantral alveolar ridge, or part of it, into the sinus, thus establishing a new sinus bottom at a higher level and creating an empty space between it and the alveolar crest. Various grafting techniques are applied at the empty space to induce new bone formation and convert it into a newly constructed ridge allowing placement of DI. The two main surgical approaches of MSFE are the lateral window (external) approach and the transalveolar (internal) approach [69].

The lateral window technique (external approach) was first presented by Tatum at the Birmingham, Alabama, implant meeting of 1976 [70]. The first publication on the technique was made by Boyne and James in 1980 [71]. The classical operation consists of the preparation of a top hinge door in the lateral sinus wall, which is luxated inward and upward together with the Schneiderian membrane to a horizontal position forming the new sinus bottom. The space below the new sinus bottom is filled with graft material. In cases with sufficient alveolar height (±4 mm) for primary stability, the DI can be inserted simultaneously with the MSFE (**Figure 5**). In cases with doubtful primary stability (bone height < 4 mm), the DI is inserted in a second procedure (**Figure 6**) when bone remodeling of the graft has taken place [1, 72].

Although safe and predictable, complications and morbidity can be associated with the lateral MSFE. Several surgical techniques have been proposed to minimize these problems with the use of specialized trephine burrs, piezosurgical devices, balloons, and hydrostatic pressure.

The transcrestal approach (internal approach) was also presented by Tatum. A "socket former" for the selected DI size was used to prepare the implant site. A green-stick fracture of the sinus floor was then created by hand-tapping the socket former towards the sinus cavity [70]. The internal approach is considered less invasive than the external lateral window approach.

The osteotome technique is a development of the transcrestal approach used for MSFE and site development by compressing the soft maxillary bone to improve the mineral density intraalveolarly by osseous deformation and trabecular microfracture [73, 74]. Summers used specialized osteotomes with increasing diameters to intrude the sinus bottom and compress the adjacent bone optimizing its density. The green-stick fractured bottom together with the sinus membrane is displaced step-by-step into the MS cavity to form a "tent" above the original sinus floor level.

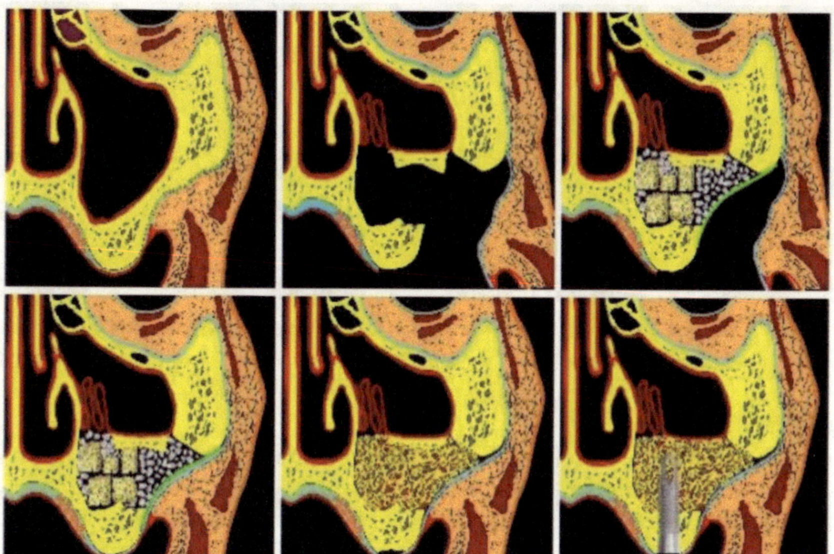

Figure 5.
MSFE with lateral approach, one-stage procedure.

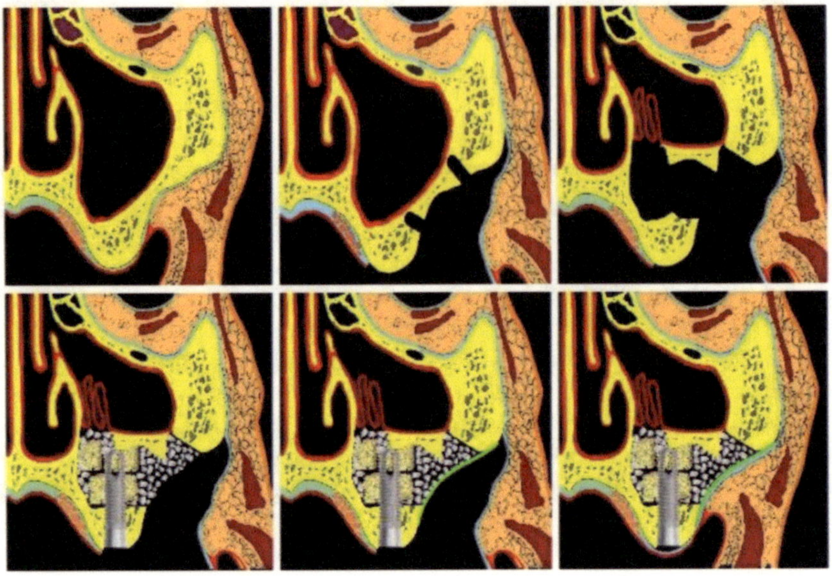

Figure 6.
MSFE with lateral approach, two-stage procedure.

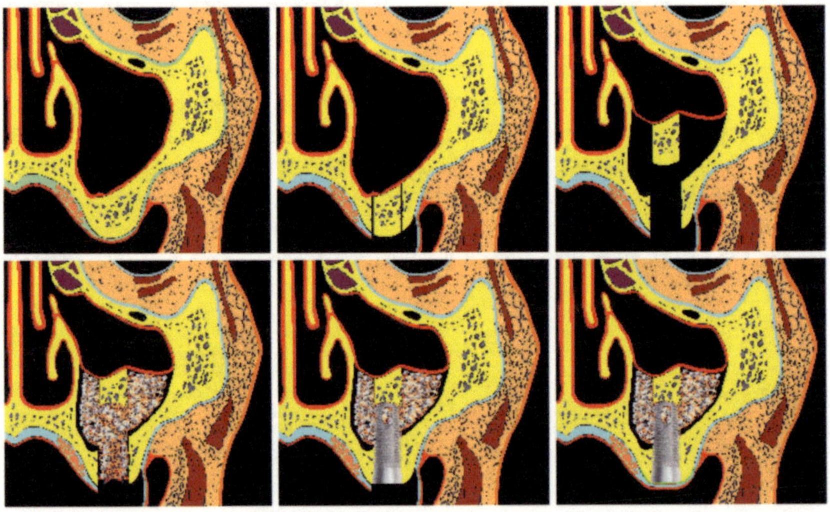

Figure 7.
MSFE with transcrestal approach, one-stage procedure.

The space within the "tent" is filled with grafting material and blood clot and the DI may be inserted into the tented space through the osteotomy opening (**Figure 7**). In cases when initial stability is doubtful the placement of the DI is postponed until the end of the healing period.

Several surgical techniques have been proposed to minimize the complications and postoperative morbidity of MSFE procedures.

Interradicular bone intrusion with MSFE is advocated in cases when sufficient in quantity (4–5 mm) interradicular septum is present after tooth removal. The central portion of the septum is freed with a standard osteotome, then a round osteotome is used to upfracture and intrude the alveolar fragment into the MS. This way, the socket is extended into the MS creating a new sinus floor at a higher level. Implant placement is carried out if adequate bone height and primary implant stability can be achieved, otherwise, the DI is inserted after a healing period of 4 months [75].

The trans-alveolar sinus elevation with ridge expansion is applicable at sites with prominent MS with horizontal alveolar resorption. The procedure combines in a single surgery MSFE with buccal ridge expansion and implant placement. The crestal distraction develops an expanded intrabony space within the cancellous bone with intact periosteal blood supply followed by immediate gentle upfracture and displacement of the floor segment into the MS [76, 77].

Other options for augmentation of the distal maxilla include:

On-lay bone grafts and MSFE. In patients with insufficient subantral bone height and unfavorable interarch relations due to advanced horizontal and vertical resorption, the MSFE procedure may be conducted simultaneously with on-lay block grafts for vertical and/or horizontal ridge augmentation. The grafting material can be harvested from extra- and intraoral donor sites or allogenous, xenogenous, and alloplastic blocks can be used [78–80].

Le Fort I downgraft with MSFE. Cases with nearly total alveolar atrophy and unfavorable maxillo-mandibular interrelations can be treated with the Le Fort I downgraft osteotomy and interpositional bone graft from the iliac crest [81–84].

Le Fort I and alveolar distraction osteogenesis with bone grafting. A moderately atrophic, retro displaced edentulous maxilla can be distracted to Class I jaw relation when combined with sinus bone grafting. When a sinus bone grafted maxilla is anteriorized via distraction osteogenesis, the repositioned sinus floor bone mass allows for axial implant development throughout the arch, especially in the canine, premolar, and first molar areas [85].

Alternative procedures were proposed to avoid the more complex MSFE surgery.

Alveolar ridge preservation is a surgical technique developed to resist postextraction ridge resorption to simplify the treatment plan for DI insertion and to decrease the need for advanced surgical procedures. Recent systematic reviews with meta-analysis confirmed the effectiveness of this approach in reducing postextraction horizontal and vertical alveolar ridge resorption when compared to spontaneous socket healing. Alveolar ridge preservation after the extraction of a maxillary molar could be regarded as a preventive treatment, in cases where a DI-supported restoration is planned, allowing a standard DI placement without additional regenerative procedures. Today alveolar ridge preservation is the most common, easy to perform, and cheap procedure aiming to control crestal bone resorption after tooth loss [47].

Other alternatives that may avoid MSFE procedures are tilted, short, zygomatic, and pterygomaxillary implants.

5. The impact of maxillary sinus anatomy on maxillary sinus elevation procedures

All MSFE techniques share common features:

- DI is inserted into the MS through an osteotomy in the sinus floor, which is presented by the subantral alveolar ridge.

- A different amount of bone from the inferior and/or the lateral sinus wall is osteotomized, drilled, or removed.

- The Schneiderian membrane alone or kept attached to an osteotomized bone segment from the MS floor and/or the lateral wall is intruded into the sinus cavity, creating the new transpositioned sinus floor.

- Under the intruded with or without osteotomized bone Schneiderian membrane an empty space ("tent effect") is created.

- The empty space is filled with bone grafts, osteoconductive or osteoinductive bone substitutes, blood cloth, different compositions with the mentioned materials or it can be left empty, to be occupied with histologically mature host bone after a corresponding healing period.

- The MSFE techniques may be applied alone or in combination with other techniques for bone regeneration and augmentation, including alveolar augmentation, grafting, and transposition, distraction osteogenesis, and free revascularized flaps.

As seen from above, the MSFE operations use the inferior and lateral MS walls to enter the sinus cavity and to reconstruct its bottom into an alveolar ridge competent enough to accept, integrate, and keep DI capable to bear masticatory loads, and to oppose alveolar atrophy.

5.1 The maxillary sinus floor

All MSFE procedures insert DI through the inferior sinus wall. The transcrestal approach with its variations uses the sinus floor to approach and elevate the Schneiderian membrane. Thus, the inferior MS wall is assigned a key role in MSFE.

The floor of the antrum in dentate adults is approximately 1 cm below the nasal floor. Anteriorly the sinus extends in general to the canine and the premolar region. There is, however, a large variety in size and shape of the sinuses even within the same person. The convex sinus floor usually reaches its deepest point at the first molar region. Roots of the maxillary teeth frequently cause convolutions in the floor of the sinus [1].

Primary alveolar bone height and width. It is believed that the concomitant actions of AA and MSP determine the bone quality and quantity of the subantral ridge. The subantral alveolar dimensions should be examined before MSFE to assure that the conditions are suitable for DI accommodation and primary stability. The prerequisites are enough height, width, bone thickness, and intermaxillary relations that permit adequate functional loading and biomechanics. These features are of crucial importance to decide whether DI can be inserted in one or a two-stage procedure. The ridge dimensions necessary for conventional DI placement are 1.5 mm of intact bone on the buccal and the palatal side to resist the horizontal AA and tension, and 2 mm above the apical tip of the implant to withstand functional loads and spare neighboring anatomical structures, if any. When planning a one-stage MSFE for an implant with a 4 mm diameter the recommended ridge dimensions must be at least 4 mm bone height and 5 mm width. The bone density must also be considered. Soft bone cannot guarantee primary stability. Otherwise, when bone quality and quantity cannot meet the needed osseous environment for a one-stage procedure, the DI should be placed in a second stage 4 to 6 months after sinus floor grafting [1]. In conclusion, when sufficient alveolar height (±4 mm) for primary stability is present, the DI can be inserted simultaneously with the MSFE. In cases with doubtful primary stability (bone height < 4 mm), the DI is inserted in a second procedure when bone-remodeling of the graft has taken place [1, 72].

Subantral dimensions as indications for MSFE procedures. The decision concerning DI size and number should rest not only on the available bone volume but should also take into consideration the prosthetic and biomechanical aspects. The classification of the International Team of Implantology categorizes the atrophic maxilla into groups, and each group requires a different surgical approach to achieve ideal bone volume and three-dimensional interarch relations. These groups are [86]:

Group 1: Insufficient subantral bone height, adequate alveolar width, acceptable vertical and horizontal interarch relations. *Surgical approach*: MSFE with bone substitute and/or autogenous bone from intraoral bone sight.

Group 2: Insufficient subantral bone height, inadequate alveolar width, acceptable vertical and horizontal interarch relations. *Surgical approach*: MSFE with horizontal ridge augmentation. Autogenous horizontal block graft (from intra- or extraoral site according to the extent of AA) may be combined with a bone substitute and barrier membrane.

Group 3. Insufficient subantral bone height, adequate alveolar width, acceptable horizontal but unfavorable vertical interarch relations due to advanced crestal resorption. *Surgical approach*: MSFE and vertical ridge augmentation. Autogenous vertical block graft (from intra- or extraoral site according to the extent of AA) may be combined with a bone substitute and barrier membrane.

Group 4. Insufficient subantral bone height, unfavorable interarch relations due to advanced horizontal and vertical crestal resorption. *Surgical approach*: MSFE with vertical and horizontal ridge augmentation. Autogenous vertical block graft (from intra- or extraoral site according to the extent of AA) may be combined with a bone substitute and barrier membrane.

More detailed classifications have been proposed by Misch [87] and Chiapasco et al. [88].

5.2 The lateral (buccal) wall and trap-door preparation

The external MSFE enters the MS by preparing a hinge trapdoor osteotomy in it which is intruded into the sinus (**Figure 8**).

The lateral sinus wall is covered by muscle-periosteal tissue, containing the facial artery and vein, the lymphatic system, and the infraorbital nerves [69, 89]. The wall usually is thin, semi-transparent and the grayish blue Schneiderian membrane can be seen through it. The thin wall facilitates door preparation and intrusion; if this is not the case, it should be thinned out to ease the mobilization of the membrane from the inner aspect of the MS. A trapdoor that follows the inner

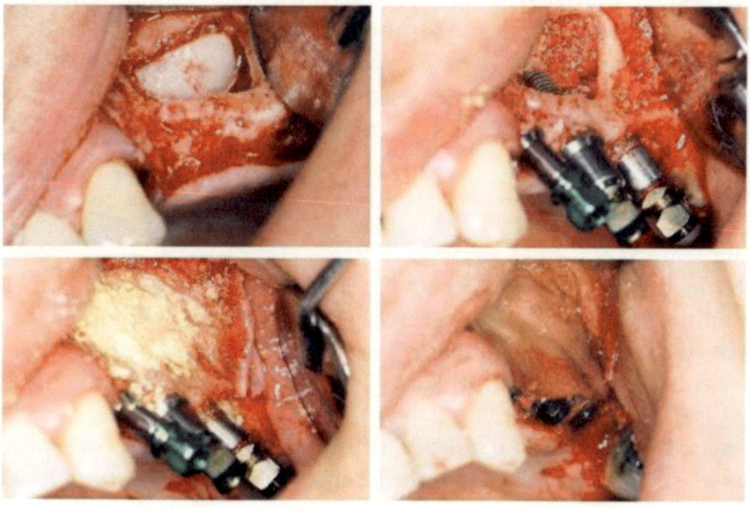

Figure 8.
Lateral MSFE, trapdoor preparation and intrusion.

shape of the MS with a wide cranial hinge base and rounded corners is advocated. Three-dimensional cone-beam computed tomography and clinical inspection will provide information on the form, the curvature, the extent, and the circumference of the sinus. The rounded corners help door mobilization and intrusion and reduce the incidence of Schneiderian membrane perforations. After the preparation of the door is finished the Schneiderian will be visualized. Normal MS anatomy will allow the trapdoor to be intruded and lifted to a horizontal position. This is possible if only the Schneiderian membrane is sufficiently mobilized from the sinus floor. The too convex outer aspect of the lateral wall (the zygomatic process of the maxilla) restricts the door base to function as a hinge because the hinge line would cause a membrane tear during door luxation. This can be avoided by the transformation of the hinged door into a hatch door; after that, the whole bone fragment can be dislocated cranially [1].

5.3 The Schneiderian membrane

Normal antral mucosa is thin (1 mm thick) and less vascular than the nasal mucosa. The ciliated respiratory epithelium transports fluids like mucus and pus towards the internal ostium. The healthy membrane is grayish blue, with traces of blood vessels. In smokers, it may be atrophic, extremely thin, and fragile even to the slightest touch. During MSFE the membrane should be kept intact to secure hermetic graft seal. Only when the whole caudal membrane is prepared free from the sinus bottom the door can be lifted to the new horizontal position; the graft material must be placed until this level. Overfilling and tension may cause necrosis of the Schneiderian membrane, loss of graft, and sinusitis [1].

The most common complication during MSFE is the Schneiderian membrane perforation (**Figure 9**). Mobilization difficulties are met in detaching it from septa, longitudinal floor rims, convolutions, and root tip expressions. Certain anatomical features such as narrow sinuses and sharp sinus opening angles have also been recognized to increase the risk of membrane perforation. Adhesions between the oral and sinus mucosa in places with totally missing alveolar bone, as well, as scars from previous MS surgery may be a contraindication for MSFE because the membrane cannot be kept intact. Small perforations located in areas where the elevated mucosa forms multiple folds usually do not necessitate treatment because the folded membrane tends to close the perforation which heals spontaneously. Larger and/or unfolded perforations need closure and must be covered with resorbable membranes and biologic glues. In cases with very large perforations, further sinus elevation should be abandoned. Re-entry might be considered 6–8 weeks after the first surgical attempt [1].

5.4 Maxillary sinus septa

Maxillary sinus septa, or Underwood's septa, complete and incomplete, arise manly from the floor but can spur from other walls. Incomplete septa divide the floor into compartments known as recesses (**Figure 9**), while complete septa may intercept the sinus into smaller sinuses (**Figure 10**). It is assumed that floor septa function as struts bearing the masticatory forces during the dentate phase of life and slowly disappear after tooth loss.

The presence of sinus floor septa determines the shape of the osteotomy. Short floor septa have no serious impact on the lateral MSFE as they cannot block the trapdoor intrusion, but the mobilization of the Schneiderian membrane is usually difficult. With high septa the door design must either follow the floor contour, outlining it in a W-shaped or any suitable form (**Figure 14**), or two trapdoors must

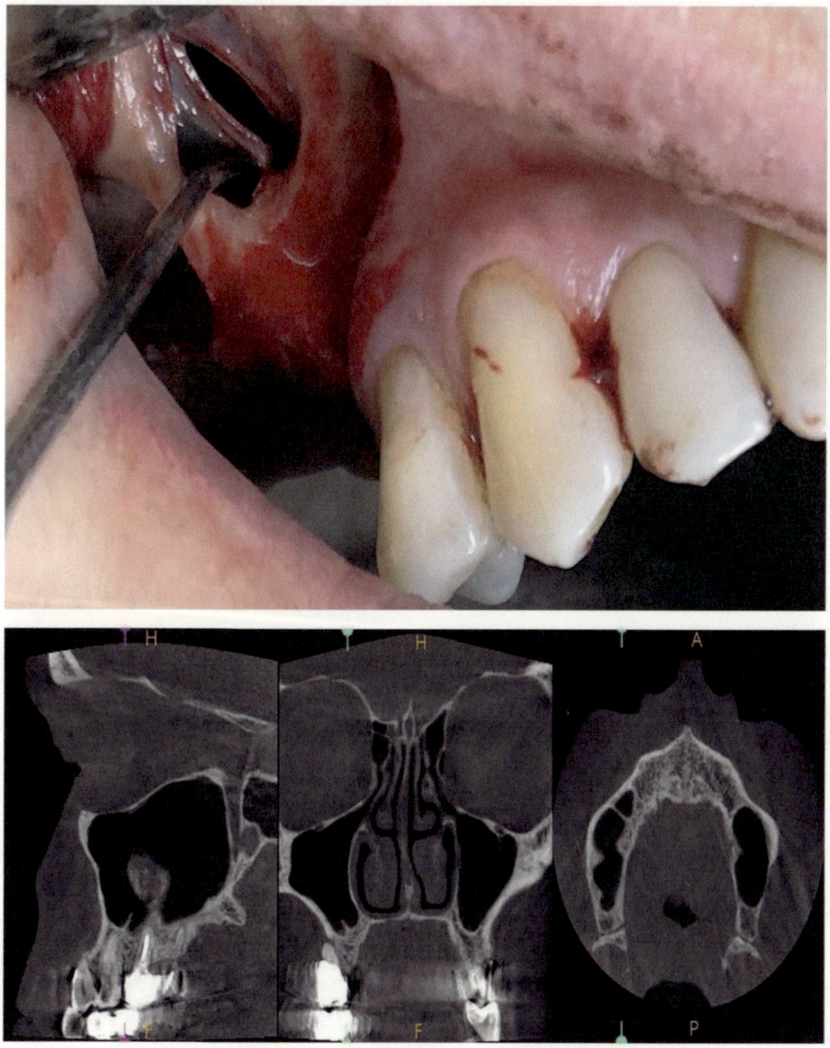

Figure 9.
A one-stage procedure consisting of extraction of the periodontally compromised right first and second maxillary molars, and lateral MSFE with simultaneous DI placement. The cause for the sinus membrane perforation is the inflammatory adhesion to the well-defined sinus floor septa and the lateral wall due to the long-lasting chronic periodontal lesions.

be performed, or the entry must be located at that side of the septum that corresponds to a recess (medial usually) in which the DI will be placed. Another option is to remove the septum through an antrostomy after the sinus mucosa has been prepared [1].

5.5 The narrow sinus

Narrow MS can only be recognized on a CT scan [90–92]. The narrow sinus, similarly, to high antral septa, will not allow for the upward intrusion of the trapdoor to the appropriate level (**Figure 11**), because the sharp MS opening angle is a predisposition to a Schneiderian membrane perforation.

The solutions to this situation are either to make an antrostomy, removing the osteotomized segment of the lateral sinus wall, or convert the trapdoor into a hatch door, mobilized all around and kept attached to the sinus membrane peduncle only.

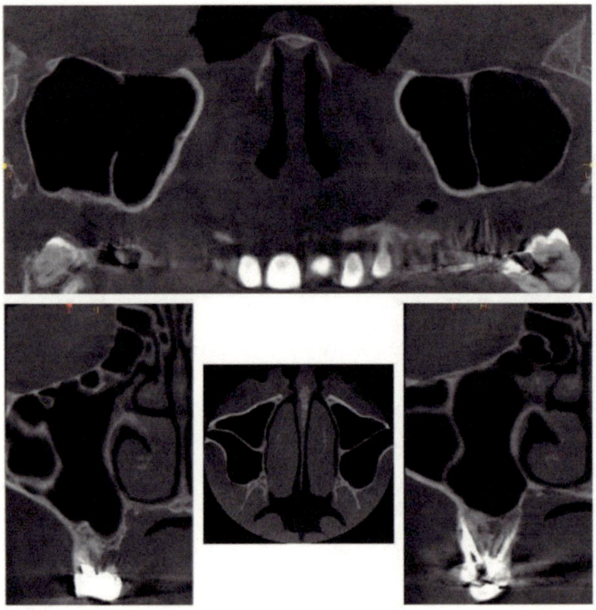

Figure 10.
Complete septa may divide the sinus into smaller sinuses.

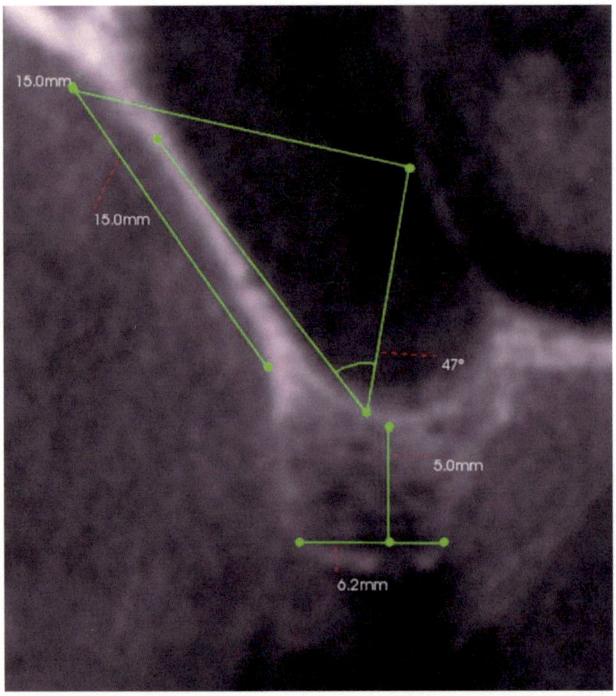

Figure 11.
The narrow sinus will not allow for the upward intrusion of the trapdoor.

5.6 Anterior (buccal) wall and the infraorbital foramen

The anterior wall is made of thin compact bone, containing the neurovascular canals to the anterior teeth if present. The structure that must be avoided cranially is the infraorbital foramen. Not only might the preparation of the door be a threat

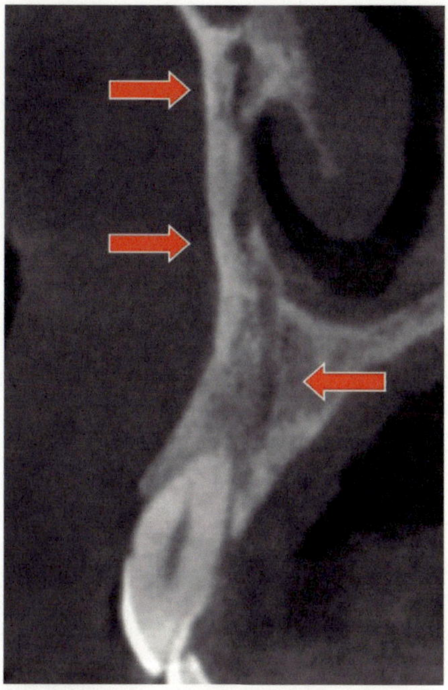

Figure 12.
Canalis sinuosus, ending in the canine area.

to the neuro-vascular bundle but also the possibility of mechanical damage by the wound retractor should be regarded. Normally however there is no reason for such high preparations because there is no need for such a high "door". It might even cause the door to be too large for the width of the sinus, making it impossible to raise it to a horizontal level. This problem may also be encountered with the combination of "normal" sized doors and very narrow sinuses [1].

Canalis sinuosus is a small canal running through the anterior wall of the maxilla and then along the lateral wall of the nasal cavity, residing in the alveolar process of the maxilla (**Figure 12**). Its nerves and vessels supply anterior teeth and adjacent soft tissues. In rare cases, the small canal could be damaged if the anterior edge projection of the trapdoor goes too far anteriorly above the first maxillary premolar [93].

5.7 The internal or nasal wall and maxillary ostium

The internal wall has a rectangular shape and forms the bony septum between the nasal cavity and MS. The inferior part of the wall corresponds with the inferior meatus of the nasal cavity, marked by the tuberosity of the inferior concha at the top. At the cranial side of this wall a fragile bony structure, the so-called sinus hiatus or ostium, can be recognized, which drains the sinus into the middle nasal meatus. The architecture of the MS drainage is complex and consists of three passages. The first one is the ostium, which leads into the second passage, the ethmoid infundibulum, that conducts mucus from the maxillary sinus into the middle meatus via the third passage, the hiatus semilunaris. The obstruction of any of the three interconnected passages may lead to retention of the sinus secretions [94]. The competence of the ostium must be evaluated before and after MSFE and kept intact because arrests on drainage during the healing period may compromise the postoperative result (**Figure 13**).

An accessory ostium may sometimes be found on the medial wall. When this occurs, it should be identified before any maxillary sinus elevation procedure is performed to avoid detaching the mucosa up to this point.

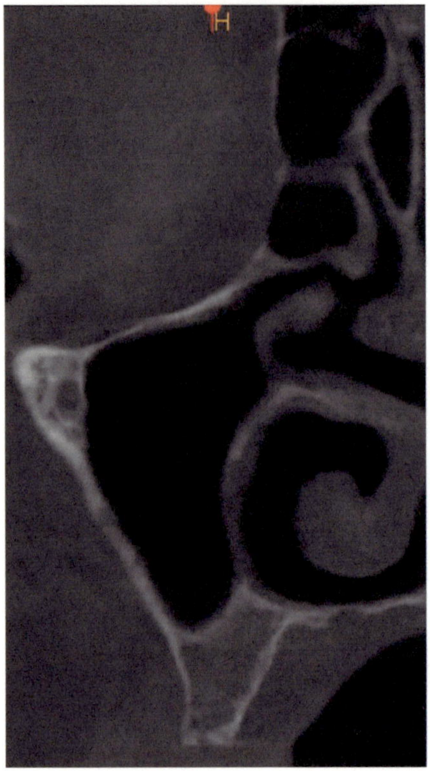

Figure 13.
Competent MS drainage.

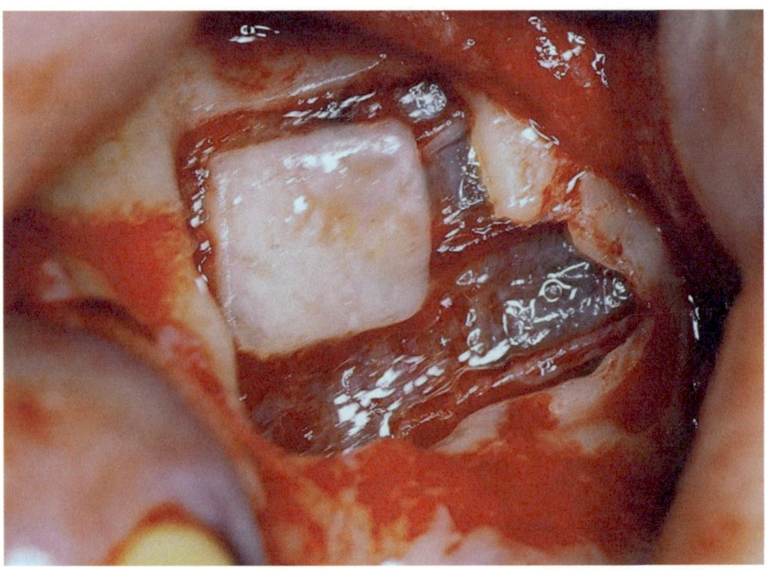

Figure 14.
Lateral MSFE with hatch door design and additionally enlarged window to follow the floor topography due to the presence of a floor septum. Note the neurovascular structures attached to the Schneiderian membrane. At the top, the membrane is traversed by the medial alveolar nerve, the bottom is crossed by the alveolar antral artery and its accompanying vein is seen in the middle.

Normal sinus physiology could be threatened if the function of the ciliated epithelium of the ostium is impaired after MSFE, but there is no clinical evidence for changed antral mucosal function after surgery [1].

5.8 Blood supply

The blood supply of the MS derives from the infraorbital artery, the greater palatine artery, and the posterior superior alveolar artery. Several anastomoses between the posterior superior alveolar artery and the infraorbital artery can be found inside the bony lateral antral wall, which also supplies the Schneiderian membrane as well as in the epiperiosteal vestibular tissues. The major intraosseous anastomosis, called the alveolar antral artery (**Figure 14**), passes through the area of the bony window [95]. In its course, the artery can lie strictly within the sinus wall, or it may occupy the inner surface of the bony window, or even may be attached to the outer

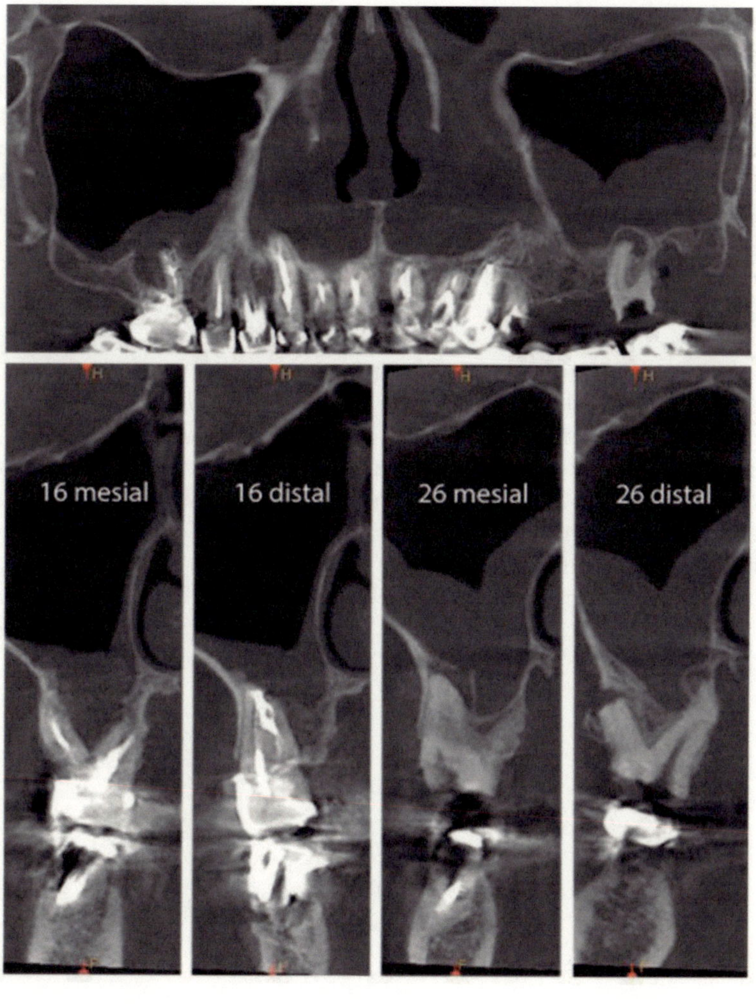

Figure 15.
Heavy chronic odontogenic sinusitis on both sides due to extensive endodontic and periodontal lesions. The interradicular septum of 16 is fully destroyed. The apical lesion around the mesio-vesibular root of 26 perforates the sinus floor and drains directly into the sinus.

aspect of the Schneiderian membrane. The mean distance between the intraosseous anastomoses and the alveolar ridge is 19 mm. The epiperiosteal vestibular anastomosis is situated at a more cranial level [1]. Hemorrhages during sinus grafting are rare since the main arteries are not within the surgical area. However, small vessels might be damaged. If they are located in the exposed Schneiderian membrane, they should best be left to stop spontaneously or stopped by slight gauze pressure. Electro-surgery will cause necrosis of the membrane and therefore can threaten the coverage of the graft.

The posterior teeth are supplied by neurovascular branches coming from the maxillary tuberosity. This must be kept in mind because a surgical approach too close to the apexes of vital neighboring teeth might devitalize them.

6. Maxillary sinus elevation and odontogenic sinus infections

Odontogenic infection of the MS, odontogenic sinusitis, accounts for about 10–25% of all cases suffering MS sinusitis. The primary cause usually is periapical or periodontal infection from maxillary molars and premolars, as the inflammatory exudate can easily erode through the thin floor to drain into the sinus (**Figure 15**). The etiology is predominantly bacterial, but, fungal infections must also be suspectedbecause filamentous fungi from endodontically and periodontally compromised teeth can invade the sinus. Such teeth can serve as reservoirs for most common fungal infections as candidiasis, aspergillosis, and mucormycosis (zygomycosis). Allergic conditions may also lead to chronic reactive mucosal changes and can block normal sinus drainage. Obstruction of the osteomateal unit is thought to be pivotal in the development and persistence of sinusitis (**Figure 15**) [96, 97].

In many patients, the disease is asymptomatic or causes minor inconveniences which explains why its role in MSFE is underestimated [97]. It must be emphasized that retention of secretions may compromise the short-term and long-term treatment success. The careful clinical and roentgenological examination is mandatory before MSFE, with no regard to the chosen approach. Chronic sinusitis is recognized as a thickening of the Schneiderian membrane and presents a contra-indication for sinus elevation. Even asymptomatic forms of infection cause serious complications. The operation should be postponed until the condition is placed under control.

Author details

Nikolay Uzunov[1]* and Elena Bozhikova[2]

1 Private Practice, Plovdiv, Bulgaria

2 Medical University Plovdiv, Plovdiv, Bulgaria

*Address all correspondence to: nouzoun.nu@gmail.com

References

[1] Bergh JPA, Bruggenkate ten CM, Disch F, Tuinzing D. Anatomical aspects of sinus floor elevations. Clin Oral Impl Res. 2000;11(3):256-265. doi:10.1034/j.1600-0501.2000.011003256.x 17

[2] Sharan A, Madjar D. Maxillary sinus pneumatization following extractions: a radiographic study. Int J Oral Maxillofac Implants. 2008;23(1):48-56.

[3] Esposito M, Felice P, Worthington H. (2014). Interventions for replacing missing teeth: augmentation procedures of the maxillary sinus. Cochrane Database Syst Rev. 2014;13(5), CD008397. doi:10.1002/14651858.CD008397.pub2.

[4] Tarun Tumar A, Anand U. Maxillary sinus augmentation. J Int Clin Dent Res Organ. 2015;7:81-93.

[5] Alveolar atrophy. (n.d). In Farlex partner medical dictionary. (2012). Retrieved 5 27, 2021, from https://medical-dictionary.thefreedictionary.com/alveolar+atrophy

[6] Schropp L, Wenzel A, Kostopoulos L, Karring T. Bone healing and soft tissue contour changes following single-tooth extraction: a clinical and radiographic 12-month prospective study. Int J Periodontics Restorative Dent. 2003;23(4):313-323.

[7] Lekovic V, Camargo PM, Klokkevold PR, Weinlaender M, Kenney EB, Dimitrijevic B, Nedic M. Preservation of alveolar bone in extraction sockets using bioabsorbable membranes. J Periodontol. 1998;69: 1044-9.

[8] Tallgren A. The continuing reduction of the residual alveolar ridges in complete denture wearers: a mixed-longitudinal study covering 25 years. 1972. J Prosthet Dent 2003;89(5): 427-435.

[9] Pinho M, Roriz V, Novaes A, Taba MJ, Grisi M, de Souza S., Palioto D. Titanium membranes in prevention of alveolar collapse after tooth extraction. Implant Dent. 2006;15(1):53-62.

[10] Hansson S, Halldin A. Alveolar ridge resorption after tooth extraction: A consequence of a fundamental principle of bone physiology. J Dent Biomech. 2012;31. doi:10.1177/1758736012456543 20

[11] Beaupre G, Orr T, Carter D. An approach for time dependent bone modeling and remodeling - theoretical development. J Orthop Res. 1990;8(5):651-661. doi: 10.1002/jor.1100080506.

[12] Frost HM. Perspectives: a proposed general model of the "mechanostat" (suggestions from a new skeletal-biologic paradigm). Anat Rec. 1996;244(2):139-47.

[13] Burger E, Klein-Nulend J. Mechanotransduction in bone – role of the lacuno-canalicular network. FASEB J. 1999;13 (Suppl.), S101-S112.

[14] Schneider P, Meier M, Wepf R, Müller R. Towards quantitative 3D imaging of the osteocyte lacuno-canalicular network. Bone. 2010;47; 848-858

[15] Bonewald L. The amazing osteocyte. J Bone Miner Res. 2011;26(2):229-238. doi:10.1007/s11914-019-00515-z

[16] Dallas S, Prideaux M, Bonewald L, et al. The osteocyte: An endocrine cell … and more. Endocr. Rev. 2013;34(5), 658-690.

[17] Weinkamer, R, Kollmannsberger P, Fratzl P. (2019). Towards a connectomic description of the osteocyte lacunocanalicular network in bone. Curr Osteoporos Rep. 2019;1:186-194.

[18] Yu B, Pacureanu A, Olivier C, Cloetens C, Peyrin F. Assessment of the human bone lacuno-canalicular network at the nanoscale and impact of spatial resolution. Sci Rep. 2020;10:4567. doi:10.1038/s41598-020-61269-8

[19] Bonewald L. Osteocytes as dynamic multifunctional cells. Ann N Y Acad Sci. 2007;1116:281-290. doi:10.1196/annals.1402.018

[20] Hamrick, M. Leptin, bone mass, and the thrifty phenotype. J Bone Miner Res. 2004;19(10):1607-1611. doi:10.1196/annals.1402.018.

[21] Nakashima T, Hayashi, M, Fukunaga T, Kurata K, Oh-Hora M, Feng JQ, et. al. Evidence for osteocyte regulation of bone homeostasis through RANKL expression. Nat. Med. 2011;17(10):1231-1234.

[22] Fulzele K, Lai F, Dedic F, Saini V, Uda Y, Shi C, et al. Osteocyte-secreted Wnt signaling inhibitor sclerostin contributes to beige adipogenesis in peripheral fat depots. J. Bone Miner. Res. 2017;32:373-384.

[23] Rauch F. The brains of the bones: how osteocytes use WNT1 to control bone formation. J. Clin. Invest. 2017;127(7):2539-2540.

[24] Asada N, Sato M, Katayama Y. Communication of bone cells with hematopoiesis, immunity, and energy metabolism. BoneKEy Rep. 2015;4:748. doi:10.1038/bonekey.2015.117.

[25] Jacobs C, Temiyasathit S, Castillo A. Osteocyte mechanobiology and pericellular mechanics. Annu Rev Biomed Eng. 2010;12(1);369-400. doi:10.1146/annurev-bioeng-070909-105302

[26] Moester M, Papapoulos S, Löwik C, Van Bezooijen R. Sclerostin: current knowledge and future perspectives. Calcif Tissue Int. 2010;87(2):99-107

[27] McDonald M, Khoo W, Ng P, Xiao Y, Zamerli J, Thatcher P. et al. Osteoclasts recycle via osteomorphs during RANKL during RANKL-stimulated bone resorption. Cell. 2021. doi:10.1016/j.cell.2021.02.0022021

[28] Qin Y-X, Rubin C, McLeod K. Nonlinear dependence of loading intensity and cycle number in the maintenance of bone mass and morphology. J Orthop Res. 1998;16:482-489.

[29] Lanyon L. Experimental support for the trajectorial theory of bone structure. J Bone Joint Surg Br. 1974;156-B(1);160-166.

[30] Skedros J, Baucom S. Mathematical analysis of trabecular 'trajectories' in apparent trajectorial structures: the unfortunate historical emphasis on the human proximal femur. J Theor Biol. 2007;244(1):15-45.

[31] Pontzer H, Lieberman D, Momin E, Devlin M, Polk J, Hallgrímsson B, Cooper, D. Trabecular bone in the bird knee responds with high sensitivity to changes in load orientation. J Exp Biol 2006;209(1):57-75.

[32] Petrtyl M, Hert J, Fiala P. Spatial organization of the Haversian bone in man. J Biomech. 1996;29(2):161-169.

[33] Cardaropoli G, Araujo M, Lindhe J. Dynamics of bone tissue formation in tooth extraction sites. An experimental study in dogs. J Clin Periodontol. 2003;30(9):809-818. doi:10.1034/j.1600-051x.2003.00366.x.

[34] Pietrokovski J. Massler M. Alveolar ridge resorption following tooth extraction. J Prosthet Dent. 1967;17(1):21-27.

[35] Botticelli D, Berglundh T, Lindhe J. Hard-tissue alterations following immediate implant placement in extraction sites. J Clin Periodontol, 2004;31:820-828.

[36] Araujo M, Sukekava F, Wennstrom JL, Lindhe J. Ridge alterations following implant placement in fresh extraction sockets: an experimental study in the dog. J Clin Periodontol. 2005;32(6):645-652.

[37] Sanz M, Cecchinato D, Ferrus J, Pjetursson EB, Lang NP, Lindhe J. A prospective, randomized-controlled clinical trial to evaluate bone preservation using implants with different geometry placed into extraction sockets in the maxilla. Clin Oral Implants Res. 2010;21(1):13-21.

[38] Rubin C, Sommerfeldt D, Judex S, Qin, Y. Inhibition of osteopenia by low magnitude, high-frequency mechanical stimuli. Drug Discov Today. 2001;6(16): 848-858.

[39] Toro-Ibacache V, Zapata Muñoz V, O'Higgins P. The relationship between skull morphology, masticatory muscle force and cranial skeletal deformation during biting. Ann Anat. 2016;203: 59-68.

[40] Van der Weijden F, Dell'Acqua F, Slot DE. Alveolar bone dimensional changes of post-extraction sockets in humans: a systematic review. J Clin Periodontol. 2009;36(12):1048-1058.

[41] Covani U, Ricci M, Bozzolo G, Mangano F, Zini A, Barone A. Analysis of the pattern of the alveolar ridge remodeling following single tooth extraction. Clin Oral Implants Res. 2011;22(8):820-825.

[42] Chappuis V, Engel O, Reyes M, Shahim KN-P, Buser D. Ridge alterations post-extraction in the esthetic zone: a 3D analysis with CBCT. J Dent Res. 2013;92(12);195s-201s. doi:10.1177/0022034513506713.

[43] Misawa M, Lindhe J, Araújo MG. The alveolar process following single-tooth extraction: a study of maxillary incisor and premolar sites in man. Clin Oral Implants Res. 2016 Jul;27(7):884-9.

[44] Covani U, Giammarinaro E, Marconcini S. Alveolar socket remodeling: The tug-of-war model. Med Hypotheses. 2020;142(109746).

[45] Noelken R, Oberhansl F, Kunkel M, Wagner W. Immediately provisionalized OsseoSpeed(™) Profile implants inserted into extraction sockets: 3-year results. Clin Oral Implants Res. 2016;27(6):744-9.

[46] Pramstraller M, Farina R, Franceschetti G, Pramstraller C, Trombelli L. Ridge dimensions of the edentulous posterior maxilla: a retrospective analysis of a cohort of 127 patients using computerized tomography data. Clin Oral Implants Res. 2011 Jan;22(1):54-61. Erratum in: Clin Oral Implants Res. 2011 Feb;22(2):235.

[47] Lombardi T, Bernardello F, Berton F, Porrelli D, Rapani A, Piloni A-C, et al. Efficacy of alveolar ridge preservation after maxillary molar extraction in reducing crestal bone resorption and sinus pneumatization: A multi-center prospective case-control study. BioMed Res Int. 2018;9352130.

[48] Adibelli ZH, Songu M, Adibelli H. Paranasal sinus development in children: A magnetic resonance imaging analysis. Am J Rhinol Allergy. 2011;25(1):30-5.

[49] Nuñez-Castruita A, López-Serna N, Guzmán-López S. Prenatal development of the maxillary sinus: a perspective for paranasal sinus surgery. Otolaryngol Head Neck Surg. 2012;146(6):997-1003.

[50] Scuderi AJ, Harnsberger HR, Boyer RS. Pneumatization of the paranasal sinuses: normal features of importance to the accurate interpretation of CT scans and MR images. AJR Am J Roentgenol. 1993;160(5):1101-1104.

[51] Hauman C, Chandler N, Tong D. Endodontic implications of the maxillary sinus: a review. Int Endod J. 2002;35:127-141.

[52] Eberhardt JA, Torabinejad M, Christiansen EL. A computed tomographic study of the distances between the maxillary sinus floor and the apices of the maxillary posterior teeth. Oral Surg Oral Med Oral Pathol. 1992;73(3):345-6.

[53] Ariji Y, Kuroki T, Moriguchi S, Ariji E, Kanda S. Age changes in the volume of the human maxillary sinus: a study using computed tomography. Dentomaxillofac Radiol. 1994;23(3): 163-8.

[54] Ariji Y, Obayashi N, Goto M, Izumi M, Naitoh M, Kurita K, Shimozato K, Ariji E. Roots of the maxillary first and second molars in horizontal relation to alveolar cortical plates and maxillary sinus: computed tomography assessment for infection spread. Clin Oral Investig. 2006;10(1): 35-41.

[55] Gu Y, Sun C, Wu D, Zhu Q, Leng D, Zhou Y. Evaluation of the relationship between maxillary posterior teeth and the maxillary sinus floor using cone-beam computed tomography. BMC Oral Health. 2018 3;18(1):164.

[56] Cavalcanti MC, Guirado TE, Sapata VM, Costa C, Pannuti CM, Jung RE, César Neto JB. Maxillary sinus floor pneumatization and alveolar ridge resorption after tooth loss: a cross-sectional study. Braz Oral Res. 2018;32:e64.

[57] Kwak HH, Park HD, Yoon HR, Kang MK, Koh KS, Kim HJ. Topographic anatomy of the inferior wall of the maxillary sinus in Koreans. Int J Oral Maxillofac Surg. 2004;33(4):382-8.

[58] Wehrbein H, Diedrich P. Die fortschreitende Pneumatisation der basalen Kieferhöhle nach Extraktion und Lückenschluss [Progressive pneumatization of the basal maxillary sinus after extraction and space closure]. Fortschr Kieferorthop. 1992 Apr;53(2):77-83. German.

[59] Nimigean VR, Nimigean V, Maru N, Andressakis D, Balatsouras DG, Danielidis V. The maxillary sinus and its endodontic implications: clinical study and review. B-ENT. 2006;2(4):167-75.

[60] Kasikcioglu A, Gulsahi A. Relationship between maxillary sinus pathologies and maxillary posterior tooth periapical pathologies. Oral Radiol 2016;32:180-186. doi:10.1007/s11282-015-0231-7.

[61] Chaiyasate S, Baron I, Clement P. Analysis of paranasal sinus development and anatomical variations: a CT genetic study in twins. Clin Otolaryngol. 2007;32(2):93-97.

[62] Butaric LN, Maddux SD. Morphological Covariation between the Maxillary Sinus and Midfacial Skeleton among Sub-Saharan and Circumpolar Modern Humans. Am J Phys Anthropol. 2016;160(3):483-97. doi: 10.1002/ajpa.22986. Epub 2016 Mar 24. PMID: 27009746.

[63] Ariji Y, Ariji E, Yoshiura K, Kanda S. Computed tomographic indices for maxillary sinus size in comparison with the sinus volume. Dentomaxillofac Radiol. 1996 Jan;25(1):19-24.

[64] Ohba T, Langlais RYM, Tanaka T, Hashimoto K. Maxillary sinus floor in edentulous and dentate patients. Indian J Dent Res. 2001;12(3): 121-125.

[65] Wagner F, Dvorak G, Nemec S, Pietschmann P, Figl M, Seemann R. A principal components analysis: how pneumatization and edentulism contribute to maxillary atrophy. Oral Dis. 2017;23(1):55-61.

[66] Nimigean V, Nimigean VR, Măru N, Sălăvăstru DI, Bădiţă D, Tuculină MJ. The maxillary sinus floor in the oral implantology. Rom J Morphol Embryol. 2008;49(4):485-9.

[67] Shahbazian M, Xue D, Hu Y, van Cleynenbreugel J, Jacobs R. Spiral computed tomography based maxillary sinus imaging in relation to tooth loss, implant placement and potential grafting procedure. J Oral Maxillofac Res. 2010;1(1):e7.

[68] Levi I, Halperin-Sternfeld M, Horwitz J, Zigdon-Giladi H, Machtei EE. Dimensional changes of the maxillary sinus following tooth extraction in the posterior maxilla with and without socket preservation. Clin Implant Dent Relat Res. 2017;19(5): 952-958.

[69] Kao D. Clinical Maxillary Sinus Elevation Surgery. (D. Kao, Ed.) 2014. Willey-Blackwell. doi:10.1002/9781118871331.

[70] Tatum H Jr. Maxillary and sinus implant reconstructions. Dent Clin North Am. 1986;30(2):207-209.

[71] Boyne P, James R. Grafting of the maxillary sinus floor with autogenous marrow and bone. J Oral Surg 1980;38: 613-616.

[72] Woo I, Le BT. Maxillary sinus floor elevation: review of anatomy and two techniques. Implant Dent. 2004;13(1): 28-32.

[73] Summers RB. A new concept in maxillary implant surgery: the osteotome technique. Compendium. 1994;15(2):152, 154-6, 158 passim; quiz 162.

[74] Summers, R. Osteotome technique for site development and sinus floor augmentation. In: Jensen O, editor. The sinus bone graft. 2nd ed. Chicago: Quintesence Publishing Co, Inc.;2006: 263-272.

[75] Fugazzotto P, Jensen *O. Sinus* floor augmentation at the time of tooth removal. In: Jensen O, editor. The sinus bone graft. 2nd ed. Chicago: Quintesence Publishing Co, Inc.;2006; 67-74.

[76] Bruschi GB, Scipioni A, Calesini G, Bruschi E. Localized management of sinus floor with simultaneous implant placement: a clinical report. Int J Oral Maxillofac Implants. 1998;13(2):219-26.

[77] Cullum D, Jensen O. Trans-alveolar sinus elevation with ridge expansion. In: Jensen O, editor. The sinus bone graft. 2nd ed. Chicago: Quintesence Publishing Co, Inc.;2006;251-262).

[78] Isaksson S, Alberius P. Maxillary alveolar ridge augmentation with onlay bone-grafts and immediate endosseous implants. J Craniomaxillofac Surg. 1992;20(1):2-7.

[79] Schwartz-Arad D, Levin L. Intraoral autogenous block onlay bone grafting for extensive reconstruction of atrophic maxillary alveolar ridges. J Periodontol. 2005;76(4):636-641.

[80] Schwartz-Arad D, Ofec R, Eliyahu G, Sterer N, Ruban A. Onlay bone graft augmentation for the treatment of maxillary atrophy: Long-term (up to 131 months) follow-up on 272 implants. Journal of Cosmetic Dentistry. 2015;31(3):78-93.

[81] Farrell CD, Kent JN, Guerra LR. One-stage interpositional bone grafting and vestibuloplasty of the atrophic maxilla. J Oral Surg. 1976 Oct;34(10):901-6. PMID: 787482.

[82] Kahnberg K, Nystrom E, Bartholdsson L. Combined use of bone grafts and Branemark fixtures in the treatment of severely resorbed maxillae. Int J Oral Maxillofac Implants. 1989:4:297-304.

[83] Isaksson S. Evaluation of three bone grafting techniques for severely

resorbed maxillae in conjunction with immediate endosseous implants. Int J Oral Maxillofac Implants. 1994;9: 679-688.

[84] Jensen O, Branca R. Le Fort I downgraft with sinus elevation. In: Jensen O, editor. The sinus bone graft. 2nd ed. Chicago: Quintesence Publishing Co, Inc.;2006;241-250.

[85] Jensen O, Laster Z. Le Fort I and alveolar distraction osteogenesis with bone grafting. In: Jensen O, editor. The sinus bone graft. 2nd ed. Chicago: Quintesence Publishing Co, Inc.;2006;281-288.

[86] Katsuyama, H., & Jensen, S. ITI treatment guide. Sinus floor elevation procedures. 1st ed. Vol. 5. (S. Chen, D. Buser, & D. Wismejer, Eds.) Berlin: Quintessence Publishing Co, Inc.; 2011.

[87] Misch, C. Treatment planning for the edentulous posterior maxilla. In: Misch, C, editor. Contemporary Implant Dentistry. St. Louis: Mosby-Elsevier; 2008: 389-405.

[88] Chiapasco M, Zaniboni M, Rimondini L. Dental implants placed in grafted maxillary sinuses: a retrospective analysis of clinical outcome according to the initial clinical situation and a proposal of defect classification. Clin Oral Implants Res. 2008;19(4):416-28.

[89] Chanavaz M. Maxillary sinus: anatomy, physiology, surgery, and bone grafting related to implantology--eleven years of surgical experience (1979-1990). J Oral Implantol. 1990;16(3): 199-209.

[90] Velloso GR, Vidigal GM Jr, de Freitas MM, Garcia de Brito OF, Manso MC, Groisman M. Tridimensional analysis of maxillary sinus anatomy related to sinus lift procedure. Implant Dent. 2006;15(2): 192-6.

[91] Cho SC, Wallace SS, Froum SJ, Tarnow DP. Influence of anatomy on Schneiderian membrane perforations during sinus elevation surgery: three-dimensional analysis. Pract Proced Aesthet Dent. 2001;13:160-3.

[92] Wagner F, Dvorak G, Nemec S, Pietschmann P, Traxler H, Schicho K, Seemann R. Morphometric analysis of sinus depth in the posterior maxilla and proposal of a novel classification. Sci Rep, 2017;7:45397.

[93] Neves FS, Crusoé-Souza M, Franco LC, Caria PH, Bonfim-Almeida P, Crusoé-Rebello I. Canalis sinuosus: a rare anatomical variation. Surg Radiol Anat. 2012;34(6):563-6.

[94] Prasanna L, Mamatha H. The location of maxillary sinus ostium and its clinical application. Indian J Otolaryngol Head Neck Surg.2010; 62(4): 335-337. doi:10.1007/s12070-010-0047-z.

[95] Valente NA. Anatomical Considerations on the Alveolar Antral Artery as Related to the Sinus Augmentation Surgical Procedure. Clin Implant Dent Relat Res. 2016;18(5):1042-1050.

[96] Ferguson M. Rhinosinusitis in oral medicine and dentistry. Aust Dent J. 2014;59(3):289-95.

[97] Selvamani M, Donoghue M, Bharani S, Madhushankari GS. Mucormycosis causing maxillary osteomyelitis. J Natural Sci Biol Med. 2015;6(2):456-459.